# Facing It

# Facing It

AIDS Diaries
and the Death of the Author

*Ross Chambers*

*Ann Arbor*
The University of Michigan Press

Copyright © by the University of Michigan 1998
All rights reserved
Published in the United States of America by
The University of Michigan Press
Manufactured in the United States of America
⊗ Printed on acid-free paper

2001   2000   1999   1998   4   3   2   1

No part of this publication may be reproduced,
stored in a retrieval system, or transmitted in any form
or by any means, electronic, mechanical, or otherwise,
without the written permission of the publisher.

*A CIP catalog record for this book is available
from the British Library.*

Library of Congress Cataloging-in-Publication Data

Chambers, Ross.
 Facing it : AIDS diaries and the death of the author / Ross Chambers.
 p. cm.
 Includes bibliographical references (p. ).
 ISBN 0-472-10958-8
 1. AIDS (Disease)—Patients—Diaries. I. Title.
RC607.A26  C4753  1998
362.1'969792—dc21          98-9005
                      CIP

> The trouble with death-at-your-doorstep
> is that it is happening to you.
> —Harold Brodkey, *This Wild Darkness*

> Death is the sanction of everything the storyteller can tell.
> He has borrowed his authority from death.
> —Walter Benjamin, "The Storyteller"

> AIDS has taught me precisely what I am writ in,
> [not water but] blood and bone and viral load.
> —Paul Monette, *Last Watch of the Night*

# Preface

Writing criticism in the midst of an epidemic can feel uncomfortably like getting on with one's needlework while the house burns down. One ought to be dialing 911, rousing sleeping children and ushering them to safety, rescuing the cat or the strongbox that holds the insurance policy and the title deed. One ought to be working with ACT-UP, hassling congress people, contributing to AIDS research. What, Eric Michaels wondered in 1988 (156–58, 106–7),[1] after reading the special AIDS issue of *October*, can criticism do? Can it fight disease, save lives?

The question was sardonic but possibly also a bit tongue-in-cheek, given that fighting the disease of AIDS and saving lives has proved difficult even for medical science. Contrary to Michaels's understandable skepticism, this essay is dedicated to the proposition that, in an epidemic, rhetoric *also* plays a not insignificant part and that the rhetorical stakes of writing an AIDS diary, as Michaels courageously did, and also of responding to it critically, are real. Why would a person at the symptomatic stage of AIDS wish to write a diary? What are the responsibilities of those who survive the diary's author as its readers? What kind of "facing up" is entailed in these practices of writing and of reading? These are what I regard as the key critical questions, and my attempt to respond to them is grounded in the observation that, when it is not possible to fight disease, save lives, or escape pain, it is still important to bear witness to that impossibility. For as Sterne, in his wry way, noticed in *Tristram Shandy*, with reference to my Uncle Toby's war wound, "the history of a soldier's wound beguiles the pain of it" (I, xxv, 79).

---

1. For readers' convenience I reference the pagination of both the Australian and the U.S. edition of *Unbecoming*, in that order.

## Preface

The reason witnessing mitigates the pain it cannot cure seems to lie in the fact that an act of witnessing, contrary to the circumstances of trauma themselves, implies a certain belief in there being a future. In a situation of extremity the desire to survive in order to tell the tale is the essential sign, whether or not that desire is requited, of a certain refusal to become a merely passive victim. In cases like that of AIDS, however, in which a certain period of survival *is* vouchsafed the writer of a witnessing text but in which the story to be told is nevertheless that of the author's dying—the story, then, of a strictly curtailed period of personal survival—a second kind of survival becomes no less essential than the first. This is the survival of the story itself, by means of which a textual subject (or "subject of writing") can pursue the task of witnessing, as a social participant, when the "writing subject" has exited the scene. But this mode of survival may well seem dubious, in exact proportion to the degree to which the curtailment of personal survival appears certain.

My essay, then, concerns the anxieties that accrue, for the writer of AIDS witness in diary form, but also for the reader of such writing, around the death of the author and the survival of the text. And since criticism has a part to play in the textual afterlife of witnessing narrative—that is, its future—part of my project consists of examining the conditions of critical responsiveness under which an essay such as my own might be considered part of a *shared* project of (always inadequate) witnessing. For as Sem Dresden has put it, concerning the experience of reading the writing of Holocaust witnesses, "taking part, in all senses of the word, becomes a possibility and a duty" (21). What I have most wanted to say, then, is finally this. First, for reading subjects as well as for writing subjects, "taking part" hinges on a willingness to "face it," without which neither mode of survival—the survival of the witness who lives to tell the story of dying, the textual afterlife (dependent on reading) of the story once told—can become a reality. But, second, facing it entails a recourse to techniques of representation, with all the conditions and consequences that representation entails, of which the first is that the act of witness can never be immediate or direct but must always be oblique and deferred with respect to its object. What we face, to put it metaphorically, we can face only in a mirror, like the ancient hero confronting the Gorgon—which means that we cannot know the "it" that we face but only write or read (it).

*Preface*

That, however, is not just the condition of AIDS witness, or of witnessing in general. It is one of the possible definitions of what is called "the human condition" itself. In light of the heavy questions and issues that lie at its horizon, my project should be understood, therefore, as a very modest one indeed. I've not attempted to cover the now vast field of AIDS witnessing in general but have simply read three diaries "written," for publication, by authors at the symptomatic stage of the disease called HIV/AIDS. I chose the diaries that made me, as their reader, feel most anxious about the fact of my readership, hoping that by looking carefully at their structures of address I might gain some insight into that anxiety and what it might mean. As it happened, two of the texts I chose were video diaries, which raised some questions about viewing as reading, but all three led me to think in the end about the sense in which reading can, and should, be understood as a practice of mourning.

I at first planned an article. It grew, as I worked on it, into the short essay that follows, in which I've retained the structure and movement of the original article, if only as a reminder of the shortfall between the issues I raise and my sketchy treatment of them. But in the context of AIDS grand statements seem particularly out of place in any case. We've watched enough public squabbles among scientific authorities and seen altogether too many press conferences called prematurely to announce supposed medical breakthroughs, and the suspicion of careerism hangs over all of us who, such as myself, have something to gain from this horrible epidemic. For reasons that I hope will become gradually clearer I believe it is important to write and to speak in response to texts of AIDS witness, and even to do so as a critic, but some of the reasons why such a response should be a chastened one have also been my concern.

The projected article from which this essay grew was in memory of my dear friend Marie Maclean, who in her life, as in her dying (not from HIV disease), set an example of how not to be a victim. An early version of chapter 5 ("Anxious Reading: Eric Michaels's *Unbecoming* and the Death of the Author") will now appear in the memorial volume *Telling Performance* being edited in her honor at the University of Delaware Press by Anne Freadman and Brian Nelson. Conversely, a short essay in *Narrative* ("Reading, Mourning, and the Death of the Author," *Narrative* 5, no. 1 [Jan. 1997]: 67–76) is based on chapter 6, as is "The Responsibility of Responsiveness: Criticism in an Age of

## Preface

Witness," *Paroles gelées* 14, no. 2 (1996, special issue): 9–27. For permission to republish I thank the editors concerned. Jean-Pierre Boulé kindly allowed me to read relevant sections of his forthcoming book *Hervé Guibert: Voices of the Self* (University of Liverpool Press). I must thank audiences at the University of Pennsylvania, Amherst College, Monash University, and the University of Western Ontario who engaged with talks closely or loosely derived from my work on *Unbecoming.* I owe an important debt to readers for the University of Michigan Press and to LeAnn Fields for their advice, and especially warm thanks are due to Anna Johnston in Australia and to my Michigan friend and colleague David Caron for their thoughtful and helpful reading of this essay. David, in particular, rescued me from more than one error. The essay is dedicated, in humility, to all who have been touched by the pain of AIDS.

# Contents

1. Writing AIDS
*1*

2. Dying as an Author
*17*

3. Confronting It: *La pudeur ou l'impudeur* and the Phantom Image
*35*

4. An Education in Seeing: *Silverlake Life*
*61*

5. Anxious Reading: Eric Michaels's *Unbecoming*
*81*

6. *RSVP*, or Reading and Mourning
*115*

Afterword
*137*

References
*143*

# I

# Writing AIDS

This is an essay about witnessing and the authority it borrows, in Walter Benjamin's stately and capacious phrase, from death. Because witnessing is mediating, we cannot say, as perhaps one might wish, and certainly not in a simple and straightforward sense, that its authority derives from the truth, itself always a mediated construct. Rather, I want to propose that it derives from the death of the author, in a sense that currently has an accustomed theoretical resonance but is also, in the case of AIDS diaries, sadly literal. I make no apology for starting with what some will feel is a theoretical detour; readers unaccustomed to theoretical concepts and exposition are asked to be patient for the space of a few pages. It will be enough to grasp the "gist" of my argument here; a degree of abstraction is the price of combining precision with economy, and my goal is to be brief.

Truthfulness, then, is itself a rhetorical product, an effect of mediation, and it entails two factors. The sentence (in Benveniste's linguistics, the *énoncé*) should be literal, and the utterance (Benveniste's *énonciation*) should be sincere. (My discourse can be literal, but if it is not also sincere [I may be self-serving, hypocritical, ironic, lying] it is not truthful; and, equally, a sincere utterance that is not simultaneously literal [I may be allegorizing or fictionalizing] cannot be truthful either.) Literality is a function of reference, a relation to the context of the sentence (what it is "about") such that the subject of the sentence is exhausted in its predication. Sincerity, on the other hand, is a relation to the context of enunciation (the circumstances in which the discourse is proffered) in which, by comparison with utterances that are, say, ironic or ambiguous or unconsciously revealing, the discourse in question exhibits zero-degree readability (interpretability): what is said exhausts what is signified.

When these two conditions are met, a third is held to be satisfied:

the conformity of the discourse, as report, to a supposedly nondiscursive actuality. This condition extends the literality of the *énoncé*, pragmatically, to the relation of the discursive to a supposedly nondiscursive world; the prestige in which it is held accounts for the long tradition by which, in witnessing (a matter in which truthfulness and lying are of the essence), an "eyewitness" account is held to be superior, as evidence (the witness was there and saw it happen), to so-called hearsay evidence, which may well be a sincere and literal report but is not "grounded in experience," that is, in some supposedly unmediated perception of the reality of things.

The veracity of witnessing thus entails sincerity, literality, and "first-handedness" of experience and report, without there being a break in the chain of testimonial factors: I sincerely report, in a literal way, what I have directly experienced. But what happens, as Lyotard (1983) asks of the Nazi gas chambers, when there are no eyewitnesses and no possibility of direct report of experience because (killed in the experience) the witnesses are dead? AIDS journals, in their turn—although they do not have the status of legal evidence, as Holocaust witness sometimes does—are similarly a form of testimonial writing whose subject is dead. In them a mortally afflicted individual (in almost every instance known to me a gay man) gives a firsthand report of the process of his own demise. But they cannot and do not, literally and sincerely, say: "I am dead." It is only in the reading situation, their context of enunciation (and so by anticipation in the writing situation), that they can *signify* "I am dead" by means of an *énoncé* (statement) that says (in brutal summary): "I am dying." "I am dying," then, is said literally (as *énoncé*) and sincerely (as *énonciation*). But when "I am dying" becomes an *énoncé* whose enunciative signification is "I am dead" (or more accurately, since the reader's point of view is determinative: "'I' is dead"), what is the status of such an utterance, one that cannot be said but only signified but on which—as in the case of the Holocaust—the whole crux of the witnessing act bears? What is at stake in witnessing when it becomes subject to reading? And what onus is on the reader upon whose act the witnessing depends, at the price of a decease?

I take it as axiomatic that sincerity, literality, and first-handedness are themselves convenient fictions. Sincerity, as a concept, is suspect if only because of the evidence of unconscious motivations (I may be sincere in saying "I love my boss," but who is to say the asseveration isn't unconsciously self-serving or a displacement of hostility?). Literality falls victim to demonstrations of the figurative status of language (with catachresis as the key figure: if the "arm" of a chair is figurative, but there is no "proper" term, who is to say that my own arm is not figurative too?). But, if sincerity and literality are dubious characteristics of discourse, it follows that no report of a nondiscursive actuality can be fully transparent or firsthand, irrespective of whether "experience" itself can be unmediated (it cannot). These are the kinds of reasons, one might surmise, that underlie Benjamin's substitution, in my epigraph, of the concept of authority for the concept of truthfulness: sincerity, literality, and first-handedness of report aren't so much the causes of discursive authority as they are its products. But what, I've often asked myself, leads him to refer to discursive authority—the authority of "telling" (*erzählen*, a cognate term)—as "borrowed from death"? This insight, poignantly relevant as it is to the telling of the AIDS story in first-person witnessing accounts, is more intuitively satisfying than it is immediately clear.

The best theoretical account of its import I can give at the present stage of my reflections is as follows. If authority is an enunciative phenomenon (a product not of speech alone but of speech in a context of enunciation), and if enunciation, therefore, cannot be directly aligned (as "sincere") on the *énoncé* (as "literal"), then there is a split between the two that can be interpreted as a gap. The split is such that it is necessary for the (grammatical) subject of an *énoncé* (whether first-person or no) to "die"—that is, to fall out of direct one-on-one relation with the enunciative situation—in order for the (interpreted) subject of enunciation to achieve, instead, authority, an authority that cannot now be a matter of veracity (a direct relation to "experience" via the referent of the *énoncé*) but, rather, one of credibility, that is, a matter of reading (a relation between two discursive subjects such that one must now produce the other through a practice of interpretation). That is, the *story told* must yield its authority (the authority of "experience" and of truth) to the *telling of the story*, a rhetorical phenomenon; and the "hero" of the narrative, let's say (whether a first-person subject or no), must figuratively "die" for the storytelling itself to attain authority as a narrational achievement. In the case of AIDS diaries the "hero" of the story told is an author, subject of the *énoncé* summarized (brutally) as "I am dying" but whose text becomes readable, in the context of enunciation, as signifying

"'I' is dead," by virtue of a realization of the *énoncé*'s prediction (either known to or surmised by the reader). The situation in which the diary is read is thus a literalization of what, according to Benjamin, as I understand him, is theoretically the case in all acts of telling: "you are no longer the hero of your own story, no longer even the narrator" (Brodkey 64). The authority of AIDS diaries is not so much "borrowed" (as a matter of theory) as it derives from the actual death of an actual author—an event on which the transformation of "I am dying" into "'I' is dead" hinges. (In this they are like the legal texts known, not coincidentally, as last "wills" and "testaments": their authority is nearly absolute, but the author can no longer participate in adjudicating their significance.)

But one might say, then, that the telling of the story *survives* the story that is told, even or particularly when that story is that of the author's demise. The author, as subject of the *énoncé* "I am dying," is offered in this way a certain mode of transfiguration or transsubstantiation, and hence of survival through an act of writing that will become readable (and enjoy authority) as a result of the author's death. For, just as it is a rule that there is no *énoncé* that is not also, and simultaneously, an enunciative act, so there is no *énonciation* that is not tied to an *énoncé:* the signification "I am dead" (in the form "'I' is dead") is available only through the vehicle of the statement: "I am dying." Thus, the act of witness performed by the readable text (as enunciation) is in part detached from, but also in part continuous with, an *énoncé* that bears witness referentially to the reality of an experience, the experience of dying and, in the case of AIDS, of a particularly distressing manner of dying. So the gap between subject of the *énoncé* and subject of the enunciation—the gap introduced by the death of the author—is not a gulf but only a split. As a result, the scenario that I find repeated, sometimes barely hinted at but at other times quite carefully developed, in AIDS diaries, notably the three I aim to read closely in this essay,[1] is a sce-

---

1. My corpus of diaries consists of: Barbedette, Dreuilhe, Duve, Fisher, Guibert 1992 and 1992a, Jarman, Joslin and Friedman, and Michaels 1990. For other important writing of AIDS witness, see Duquénelle, Guibert 1990, 1992, 1992b; Monette 1990, 1994; Wojnarowicz. I wish to thank David Caron for his invaluable help in identifying and locating certain of these texts, Jean Mainil for introducing me to Pascal de Duve's *Cargo Vie,* and John Frow for pointing me toward Jarman's *Modern Nature.*

nario of survival, which I interpret as survival *across the split* that separates the statement "I am dying" from the readable utterance " 'I' is dead."

In this scenario the recourse to writing (or, since two of the diaries are in video form, to technologies of representation), that is, the act definitional of an author—and more specifically the recourse to writing in the form of autobiography, the autobiography of a dying—functions, as it were, prophylactically. On the condition of the death of the author (as subject of the *énoncé*) something is preserved from the effect of death: an occasion of survival is offered and even a mode of posthumous action, through the authority a text can enjoy, by virtue of its readability, "beyond" the extinction of its author. Beyond the author's death as in *following* that death (writing outlives the writer) but also as its *consequence*, since reading is predicated on the unavailability of authorial authority, as controlling agent of textual meaning, and on the substitution of a form of authority that is predicated on interpretability, and so, as Benjamin says, is borrowed from death. Writing is prophylactic in this sense because it combats death, although it does so at the price of a transformation of authority—from that of truthfulness to that of credibility—that is itself predicated on the author's demise.

I'll come to another sense in which the writing of AIDS diaries is prophylactic later (see chap. 2).

As witnessing discourse, AIDS diaries challenge some conventional understandings of both the diary form and the genre of autobiography. A diary explicitly and openly conceived with a view to publication—having publication as its essential finality—does not exclude the practice of intimate self-analysis associated with the *journal intime*, but it radically changes its orientation and significance by questioning the public-private dichotomy by virtue of which the "personal" diary is defined. And an autobiography that gives priority to a witnessing impulse over the memorializing function—the retrospective construction of a "life" in its narrative configurations that might be thought characteristic of classical autobiographies—seems a departure from the genre's defining origins, while, finally, the immediacy of reporting and the episodicity of form that AIDS diaries (like other diaries) espouse simultaneously distinguish them formally from the narratives of witness, such as Holocaust accounts or *testimonios* from Central America, that have been the object of most recent critical attention.

We might wish, though, to reconsider the nature of autobiography in light both of autobiographical narratives of witness and of the witnessing orientation of AIDS diaries. It may simply be an error of perspective that leads us to read autobiography in the register of memory when the classics of the genre—Augustine or Rousseau, for example—wrote autobiographical texts that are only in part memorializing and in fairly large part also about standing up to be counted. And if memory is recruited in the autobiographical constructions of "myths to live by," as Marie Maclean puts it, the same author points out that these are in essence indistinguishable from the "myths to die by" one might wish to associate with acts of witness. For memory is as much a response to forgetting, existential complexity, and the effects of time as witnessing seeks to overcome the fact of trauma and death, and memorializing autobiography, setting out to answer the question: what did this life mean? can easily stumble on more refractory questions (what was it like, how did it feel, to live my life? what pain has it entailed?) that are closer to testimonial. Meanwhile, witnessing writing, for its part, is constantly and symmetrically brought up against a problematics of memory, if only because the attempted representation of pain entails acknowledgment of its impossibility: trauma interrupts all continuity and coherence; it challenges discursive treatment because it inhibits memory and produces amnesia. Witnessing narrative and memorializing narrative both seek, then (albeit with different emphases, perspectives, and orders of success), to create coherence and sense out of discontinuity, incoherence, and disintegration.

That said, and these affinities being acknowledged, AIDS diaries are "nonnarrative texts" of autobiographical witness because in them the retrospective orientation of memory, the question: what did this life (or these events) mean? and the need to construct significance through discursive ordering are far less urgent than a need to answer the question: how does it feel to be dying of AIDS? and a desire to make available to others, with some directness, the sense of disintegration the experience entails. For the narrative syntax of beginning, middle, and end they thus substitute the structure of chronicle, with its greater immediacy: a simple *taxis* (arrangement) of now this, now that—a contiguous rather than a cohesive series of dated "entries" having the loose character of a list. They do so for obvious reasons having to do with respect for the dailiness to which the severely ill are condemned (the simple wisdom of "taking each day as it comes") as well as acknowledgment of the impossibility of closure that stems from the disease's notorious unpredictability (in all respects other than its final outcome). But the diary form relates also to a sense of the necessary open-endedness of the witnessing project, understood as the acknowledgment of trauma, of life's refractoriness to ordering, narrativizing, and sense-making gestures: it defers and delays the responsibility of making sense, transmitting it onward in a way that has been poignantly described by Felman and Laub. AIDS journals are thus not oriented retrospectively, like the *énoncé* of classical autobiography and even "narrative" texts of witness; they look forward as enunciations to a future in which they will be read, and the open-endedness of their chronicle structure implies this prospectivity as much as the thematics of survival does.

Such diaries always come to an end, of course, but they do so without concluding: there is just a final entry, followed by a white space (and usually, in front- or backmatter, an account of the author's death). Thus, their end, in spite of the author's death that it signifies, remains *suspended*, as if another entry were always possible and as if to propose, therefore, some possibility of continuation. The effect, as a result, is not unlike that of a relay, and it has something in common, therefore, with the narrative structure of relay that is characteristic of the genre of AIDS narrative that might be called "dual autobiography," in which—Paul Monette's trilogy is an instance—the writer who records another's death from AIDS is himself infected and may go on to record his own living out of the same scenario. This is the structure of Tom Joslin's video diary, *Silverlake Life*, which was finished by Peter Friedman but concerns both the death of Tom Joslin and the ailing survivorhood of his lover Mark Massi (see chap. 4). And the relay effect is explicit in Bertrand Duquénelle's *L'Aztèque*, in which the author writes, on the death of Jean-François, "A. Mon. Tour. [My. Turn. Now.]" (49).

In AIDS journals "Your. Turn. Now." or "Over. To. You." is the implicit message for the reader whenever the suspension of a diary on its author's death is perceived to transmit an obligation to continue the work of witness, work that is begun by the author as a matter of writing but, interrupted by death, requires realization if not completion through an act of reading, the nature and quality of which is thus crucial. The very first effect of a textual authority derived from (the author's) death is thus to transmit a responsibility and, as it were, an obligation, and the fact that a reader may perceive this relay structure of address, inherent in the diary's open-ended incompleteness, as a metaphorical passing on of infection is surely not accidental. A virus *has* been transmitted: not HIV but the virus of writing and reading as what I called a prophylactic practice with respect to death and as a mode of confrontation, therefore, with what cannot rightly be either said or contemplated. "How can one understand something about *death* unless they really die?" asks David Wojnarowicz (217). The relay of writing by reading, across and beyond the brute ungraspable fact of death, bears witness to a desire somehow to understand, or to make significant, the phenomenon that interrupts all intelligibility and all possibility of comprehension and structures witnessing, therefore, as the transmission of an obligation to face the fact of death and so to fail in one's responsibility even as one accepts it.

The (mediated) immediacy of the AIDS diary but also its "suspended" dependency on reading and the relay structure of its witnessing suggest a sense in which it may be fruitful, especially in view of the use of video technology in Guibert's *La pudeur ou l'impudeur* and Joslin's *Silverlake Life*, to relate the diary form to the mode of televisual broadcasting known as the "live."[2] I would argue that the category of the live is defined as much by a certain self-consciousness with respect to the technology of representation as by its relation to the living: it is the fact of its being represented, per medium of the camera, that turns the living into the live, suggesting therefore—according to a venerable if logocentric understanding of technologies of representation—that in the live the living has undergone a process of "reduction" (e.g., of three dimensions to two) that identifies repre-

---

2. What, one might ask (assuming what is itself a dubious proposition: that a written diary is easily recognized), constitutes a "video diary"? In what follows I assume, in addition to the effect of liveness (which does not preclude editing), three criteria: two on the plane of *representation*, an autobiographical relation between the holder of the camera and its object, a structural preference for chronicle grammar (discontinuous, episodic structure) as opposed to story grammar, and some *generic* reference, through setting or by quotation, for example, to "home movies" (or another indicator of domestic, intimate and/or personal discursive register). These three criteria distinguish diary from documentary, with which witnessing diaries share an informational project.

sentation as a mortifying process, in the etymological sense of that term, and endows it, therefore, with an authority "borrowed from death." AIDS journals thus not infrequently associate the fact of representation with the wasting of the body produced by the effects of disease, figuring the former by the latter while suggesting, in an extension of the metaphor, that living with AIDS is less like *living* than, as an existence already marked by death, it has the "reduced" characteristics of the live. Eric Michaels, the author of *Unbecoming*, thus writes of AIDS sardonically as a slimming process, or "cosmic personal reducing plan" (98/57). But representation is also the means whereby, through the possibility of reading it opens up, a dying subject can anticipate the possibility of a certain form of textual survival, the condition of which is, as we've seen, the death of the author; so the live, understood now as a representation that implies—as all mediation does—readability and so an orientation toward readership, can thus come to figure something like the *condition of survival* that determines the AIDS diary's ability to prolong its act of witnessing beyond the author's demise.

Yet the live is also defined—and from this it derives its effect of immediacy and spontaneity—not only in opposition to the living but also in opposition to the formal perfection of the "canned." The marker of the live thus tends to be a certain proneness to accident and error. This may be due to the incursions of the natural into the live as a performance, in the form of technical hitches, fluffed lines, and botched business (even disasters, such as the interruption of a televised baseball game by the San Francisco earthquake some years ago). Or it may—as it does in a surprising number of instances—arise from the accidental (or sometimes perhaps, not so accidental?) foregrounding of the technology of representation itself: cameras, crew, trailing cables, banks of lights, or microphone booms caught in the frame of the image. The live can thus be said to cultivate a certain kind of "messiness" as the very sign of its liveness, and this messiness can again be read polyvalently, functioning simultaneously as a figure of disorder, entropy, and communicational "noise" (and, so, a signifier of death), as a marker of the live's privileged relation, as mediation, to the living, and, finally, as a factor of readability resulting from informational complexity, self-reflexivity, and—in Paulson's sense—"noise in the channel," a readability that signifies survival. Thus, Pascal de Duve records in *Cargo Vie* (84) that he never rereads what he writes and is aware of making many contradictory statements—but he lets them stand. And in *Unbecoming* Eric Michaels (who edits his writing carefully) develops a theory of tidiness, epitomized by the hospital, as the social order that is killing him and thus implies that the looseness and disunity of the diary form—its lack of formal cohesion—is part and parcel of an overall tactics of untidiness as a mode of resistance to the forces that would like to tidy AIDS patients, gay men (and members of other stigmatized "risk groups"), out of sight, out of mind, and out of existence. It is part, that is, of a project of survival.

As for the video journals, both Guibert's *La pudeur ou l'impudeur* and Joslin's *Silverlake Life* have qualities reminiscent of home movies, a genre Guibert specifically quotes. They are shot in rooms that have a lived-in look, ranging from the incipiently untidy in Guibert's apartment to the frankly cluttered appearance of the Silverlake house, rooms that therefore contrast markedly, and significantly, with the sterility and coldness of doctors' offices and hospital equipment (which nevertheless share with the lived-in spaces a quality that makes it impossible to refer to them simply as "settings" or decor). Unexpected objects sometimes invade the frame: most memorably, perhaps, in *Silverlake Life* a cat is curled, comfortably snoozing, on the very ordinary (not hospital style) double bed in which Tom Joslin lies dying. Camera technique is quite rudimentary in *La pudeur ou l'impudeur*, and in *Silverlake Life* it is professionally informed but supremely casual: video equipment and the practices that pertain to it are foregrounded, both intentionally and accidentally, but treated always with a kind of artisanal informality. They display the video's own thoughtfulness about its status as representation, a thoughtfulness that is made even more explicit in Guibert, but they do so as part of the everyday of Silverlake life, with again a contrast with respect to the technologically impressive, but scary, CAT scan equipment (another mediator of vision) that we see in operation at the beginning of the video. It's as if the authors are using what comes to hand, the skills and equipment they happen to have, and using it in a semi-improvisational way—as a Certeauesque *art de faire,* or "making do"—in response to an emergency: a life crisis that, like a personal San Francisco earthquake, makes it an immediate and urgent necessity to find the means of witness but also of survival.

Writing AIDS

The category of the live, and in particular the immediacy of its representation of the author's dying, brings me now to what is arguably the central trope of AIDS diaries, and perhaps of AIDS writing in general. This is the trope that identifies the physical symptoms of AIDS (and most particularly the visible lesions of Kaposi's sarcoma) as writing— the writing of the AIDS-infected body, of which the authorial writing of the diary, as verbal text, is a sort of more or less direct transcription. There are next to no diaries of seropositivity;[3] it is with the onset of symptoms that the emergency becomes palpable and authors turn to their cameras and word processors and start a journal. That this connection between the appearance of symptoms and the writing of a journal is overdetermined seems obvious, and I shall return to the point, but one important way in which it is significant lies in underscoring the sense of equivalence between AIDS, as the writing of the body, and the textual production whose agent is the author—the author whose death is announced by his passage from the asymptomatic stage of positivity to the symptoms that indicate a diagnosis of AIDS. Thinking of the inscription on the tomb of Keats, Paul Monette writes: "AIDS has taught me precisely what I am writ in, blood and bone and viral load" (1994, 114); and, addressing the virus, Pascal de Duve writes (13): "VIH, c'est un peu toi qui écris ici [HIV, it's pretty much you who are doing the writing here]." (The gesture of turning over authorial authority to one "borrowed from death" is palpable in this last quotation.) In turn, the opening lines of *Unbecoming* identify KS lesions as linguistic units ("morphemes") and cast the author as one whose role is to be their interpreter, "stringing them together" into sentences that form a narrative:

9 September 1987

I watched these spots on my legs announce themselves over a period of weeks, taking them as some sort of morphemes, arising out of the strange uncertainties of the past few years to declare, finally, a scenario. As if these quite harmless look-

---

3. The (partial) exception being Jarman 1994: *Modern Nature* is a gardening diary started in, presumably, symbolic response to seropositivity, which becomes an AIDS diary in its later pages. (The early part of Gary Fisher's diary, in *Gary in Your Pocket*, might also be regarded as a seropositivity diary.)

ing cancers might, when strung together, form sentences which would give a narrative trajectory, a plot outline, at last to a disease and a scenario that had been all too vague.

(Michaels 23/3)

It's important, perhaps, to stress that the trope of "the writing of AIDS" as a figure that blurs into some sort of identification the writing of the body and the authorial text is just that: a trope, a figure. The writing of AIDS is a product of representational practices of writing *tout court*, and the body itself, although it is discursively significant, does not write. For that reason in my readings of *La pudeur ou l'impudeur*, *Silverlake Life*, and *Unbecoming* (chaps. 3, 4, and 5, respectively), I will be focusing on representations of the body in each text and taking the body not as an agent of writing on its own behalf but as a vehicle of textual self-figuration, a figurative means whereby texts indicate their enunciative situation as objects of reading, according to understandings that have been elaborated in some of my previous work (Chambers 1984, 1991, 1993). But this trope is nevertheless essential, for two related reasons. One is that it suggests a degree of complicity between the dying writers and the AIDS that is inspiring their writing: "Minuscules petites bestioles [tiny beasties]," Duve writes affectionately in addressing the virus (13), and a refrain of "Sida mon amour [AIDS my beloved]" runs through his book. Why this complicity? Against what forces is it formed? The other reason is that, as the quotation from *Unbecoming* makes clear, the writing of AIDS entails a *scenario*, "a narrative trajectory, a plot outline." Although Michaels is unspecific here about the narrative he foresees, it is hard to imagine that it might be any other scenario than that of the death of the author, presupposing the survival of textual authority that the author's death entails. It is as if the transcription of the writing of the author's body that is AIDS into the textual form of the diary represents a kind of relay operation that provides an initial model for the scenario of survival—a myth to "live by" as well as to "die by"—on which the text itself will rely in its appeal to be read. For the writing of the body will die with the body but survive in the writing of the diary.

There is another scenario of the death of the author, however, to which the trope of the writing of AIDS is also highly germane. This is a scenario not of survival beyond death but of death itself as a kind of grandiose apocalypse, or, in Duve's term, a "flamboyancy" like that of the setting sun. In the corpus of AIDS diaries known to me, Duve's *Cargo Vie* is clearly the locus classicus of this alternative myth, but this text itself has its roots in a long history of French thinking about the concept of *écriture*. In Artaud, most notably, the writing of the body as a kind of affective athleticism is a major figuration of the desire for there to be a writing not subject to the constraints of discursivity, of linguistic interchange, and the ideological construction of personhood, and Artaud's corporeal writing has migrated, more recently, both into Hélène Cixous's understanding of *écriture féminine* as "writing with the body" and into Deleuze and Guattari's elaboration of the "body without organs." In this tradition writing is understood as a vehicle of sublimity—of transcendence, rapture, and what Bataille calls "sovereignty"—more than it is concerned with readability or the desire for continued social participation beyond the author's disappearance.

It is not that Duve is not conscious of his text's witnessing function and of its relation to the discursive authority that derives from death: he writes specifically that "Ceci est un testament—au sens étymologique, un témoignage [This is a last will and testament—etymologically, a testimonial]" (46), and at one particularly striking moment he notices that the word *survie* (*survival*) is a near anagram of *virus* (14). But he is more conscious of the privileges of insight, sensitivity, and intensity of sensation accorded his dying self than he is attentive to the very real suffering (which he fully acknowledges and records) of the AIDS-infected body, and he is less anxious about the survival through reading of a textual subject than he wishes to demonstrate in the process of his disappearance a certain form of heroism:

> Regarder la mort en face sans baisser les yeux, mais au contraire en les gardant plus ouverts que jamais, mélange de défi et d'émerveillement, voilà peut-être une modeste mais authentique forme d'héroïsme, un héroïsme de poche auquel en toute humilité [. . .] j'aspire. (15)
>
> [To look Death in the face, not only with open eyes but with eyes more open than ever, with a mixture of defiance and

wonderment—perhaps there's a modest but genuine form of heroism in that, a pocket-sized heroism that in all humility I aspire to. . . .]

Words like *wonderment*, phrases like "with eyes more open than ever," signal a somewhat grandiose philosophical and aesthetic project behind the vocabulary of humility, and in fact Duve is contrasting his "héroïsme de poche"—not accidentally reminiscent of a famous paperback series, in which his diary is now published—and contrasting it favorably, as the heroism of writing, with public, socially oriented heroism, which he calls "zeroism."

The pattern of AIDS is different for every sufferer, and in Duve's case the symptoms declared themselves at an already advanced stage, through evidence that the virus had crossed the blood-brain barrier and was already in the process of destroying his brain cells. There is thus something almost literal in his belief that it is the virus, not he, that is doing the writing: "Minuscules petites bestioles, liguées par millions, vous occupez mon cerveau et vous vous en occupez. Mais avec quelle flamboyance! [Tiny beasties, banded together by the million, you're occupying my brain and taking good care of it. But how flamboyantly you do so!]" (13). The flamboyancy of the writing in *Cargo Vie*, its romantic style but more particularly the luxuriantly proliferating wordplay and punning that largely elude translation, is adduced simultaneously as evidence of the invasion of Duve's brain, its investment by parasites, and as a demonstration of Duve's contention that the ordeal of dying by AIDS is not necessarily a completely negative experience, or, as he writes in a brilliant portmanteau word that signifies both ordeal (*épreuve*) and appalling, something completely "éprouvantable" (64). Invoking the French sense of the word *parasite*, in which it refers to interference or static, "noise" in the channel of communication, we can say that AIDS is celebrated in *Cargo Vie* ("Sida mon amour") as productive of a language that is itself, like Duve's brain, richly *parasité*, a writerly language traversed by multiple effects of signification that are not necessarily compatible or reducible to the consistency that permits coherent interpretive reading. The point, indeed, is rather to *block* such recuperative reading—for example, by allowing contradictions to stand—with a view to transforming the disintegration of sense into a certain flamboyancy of signification and to substituting for the production of readability that of a certain sense of awe.

Many writers of AIDS witness have moments in which they praise AIDS or receive it as a gift, and Duve is in this respect exemplary. The myth of the "writing of AIDS" as the subjection of authorial authority to the writing of the body is a version of something that has been celebrated, especially in France, since Mallarmé: the death of the author as the subjection of authorial agency to the production of textual effects. But there is a significant difference of emphasis between Duve's insistence on authorial dying as a moment of flamboyancy in its own right and the orientation of the written AIDS body toward reading that is characteristic of the diaries whose collaboration with AIDS as an act of witness has a more immediately political sense, notably the work of Guibert, in France, as well as of English-speaking writers such as those I address in this essay. In this respect Michaels—who, beyond his initial acknowledgment of the trope of the writing of AIDS, situates AIDS as the enemy, or as a manifestation of the enemy to be opposed through writing—is (with Dreuilhe) at the opposite end of a certain spectrum from Duve and his "Sida mon amour." But Michaels shares with Guibert and with Joslin also the combination of a more trivial sense of the "messiness" and disintegration entailed by living with AIDS—the messiness that I associated with the live and with the dailiness of journal writing—with a mode of heroism that, without being zeroism, refers less to an ultimately impersonal "sovereignty" than it has to do with stoicism and defiance and the refusal to be a social victim, an attitude less oriented toward wonderment and a sense of the sublime than toward witnessing in a historical here and now and on into a textual future that will survive the death of the author.

The political meaning of this emphasis that is shared by Guibert, Joslin, and Michaels derives, I believe, from an act of choice: the decision (sometimes explicit, sometimes implied) to live with AIDS and to bear witness to the ordeal it entails, in preference to the temptation of a fast and relatively easy death, through suicide—a death that is, of course, appealing but for gay men always open to homophobic (mis)interpretation, as a sign of self-hatred. Facing down that temptation, I'll suggest in the next chapter, is a matter of facing up to the social reality of homophobia (including one's "internalized" homophobia), and doing so provides, as I'll try to demonstrate in later chapters (especially in chap. 3, on Guibert), a first model of the textual *dépassement* of death, whose scenario will then be repeated, in a new mode, in the writing of witness itself, as a bid for the survival and continued social efficacy of a certain textual subject.

But this means that ultimately it is necessary to read all AIDS diaries—the very existence of which signifies the choice to *live one's death* and to write it, as an alternative to throwing in the towel, and which are always marked by the author's consciousness of the homophobic context of their enunciation—as profoundly and deliberately political acts. They all signal a refusal on their author's part—and this is as true of Duve, in his way, as it is of the other authors—to play the role of *victim* that is marked out for AIDS patients. Their oppositionality espouses a certain way of dying and of bearing witness to that dying, one that is anything but easy, as a response, and a reproach, to those who, at the best of times, would like to see gay people (as well as the members of the other so-called AIDS risk groups) just give up and disappear. Autobiographical writing more oriented to the open-endedness of witness than to memory, an aesthetic of the live that espouses the living while inviting the "relay" of reading, a discourse of the body whose very disintegration is productive of further signification: these are the formal markers in such texts of something that is much more of the order of the political than of merely aesthetic choice, a refusal to give in and a willingness, to that end, to recruit the authority that only death, alas—the death of the author—can confer.

2

# Dying as an Author

If so, and the political context is relevant, we can now return, from another angle, to the complicity of AIDS writing in general, and the AIDS diary in particular, with the calamitous disease to which it simultaneously bears witness. Given the direness of the syndrome, such writing—the "writing of AIDS"—can only be understood as (a) an attempt to represent the syndrome's effects in the immediacy of their direness so as (b) to emphasize the significance of a choice to live with AIDS, to write it and to undergo an author's death, in preference to an alternative that is regarded as worse: the choice of witnessing over victimhood. (AIDS changes fast, as both a medical phenomenon and a social one. My reader is asked to bear in mind that, writing in 1995 and sketching the context of diaries dating from the late 1980s and early 1990s, what I describe here is a version of AIDS that will have been significantly modified by the time this essay is published. For example, no writer in my corpus could have access to or any inkling about the possibility of combination therapy.)

HIV/AIDS is not the only dire visitation the twentieth century has known. But it is a new one: time has not dulled our sensitivity to it, nor have we yet fully measured its severity, perhaps. And, in addition to its being hard to bear in itself, it afflicts populations that are historically disadvantaged: in the Third World, recently decolonized countries, and in the West—along with a few tendentiously labeled "innocent victims"—members of socially underprivileged and/or stigmatized groups: minority groups, IV drug users, hemophiliacs, gay men. The affliction of AIDS thus tends to entail the proverbial double whammy: it is a serious disease with a fatal prognosis, and the patient simultaneously lives a social and political nightmare that can have various names, among them underdevelopment, poverty, prejudice, moralism, and homophobia. For the United States David Wojnarowicz made that nightmare his literary territory, but it is not accidental that the perspective of AIDS witnessing internationally has been overwhelmingly that of middle-class, white, gay males, the only group sufficiently empowered to be able to write, and to publish, amid the daily struggle to survive.[1] AIDS witness thus falls, for good and for ill, under the category of gay writing, and homophobia is consequently its privileged target.

Death from AIDS, as these writers portray it, is slow and far from easy. After the long wait of seropositivity the symptomatic stage can come almost as a relief—until it turns out, as Michaels puts it, that AIDS is "the disease of a thousand rehearsals." "You don't die, at least right away" (139). The sequence of sudden, largely unpredictable medical emergencies and long, slow convalescences, the waiting for test results and their interpretation, the rumors of therapeutic breakthroughs, the often incautiously optimistic announcements regularly followed by disappointing outcomes (in part the subject of Guibert's *A l'ami qui ne m'a pas sauvé la vie*)—all these make AIDS (and remember I am talking here of those who can *get* medical treatment) an emotional torment as well as a physical ordeal. The opportunistic diseases are damaging, disfiguring, humiliating, and life impoverishing; they range from the indignities of diarrhea and the itch of shingles to blindness and dementia, and their treatments can be toxic as well as dispiriting. For many, contact with the institutions of modern medicine, not to mention other bureaucratic monsters, is a trauma in itself. Meanwhile, people who are themselves facing death may undergo multiple bereavements, or they may die alone, more or less

---

1. Of course, it is not simply that middle-class gay men have advantages of education, time, and access to publication. As middle-class men, they tend to experience HIV disease and the onset of AIDS as a unique visitation disrupting an otherwise comfortable life, whereas more disadvantaged people—say a woman with children living in an urban ghetto and dealing perhaps with drug problems and/or an abusive companion—experience it, in a life already defined as burdensome, as simply an additional burden. (Thus, World War I witnessing was largely done by the officer class, the rank and file having been partly inured to the conditions of trench warfare by those they endured in peacetime industrial employment.) Finally, too, it is worth pointing out that, of all the groups most directly affected by AIDS, gay males are the only ones whose intellectuals have been massively infected. For that reason first-person AIDS witnessing—as opposed to documentary reporting and the "as told to" mode prevalent in Central American testimonial—tends to be largely a gay practice of AIDS writing.

estranged from their families and with the support of only a handful of friends and ad hoc beneficent organizations.

But on top of all that, then, there are also the large-scale social factors to deal with, the other part of the whammy. In underdeveloped countries and urban ghettos in the United States large numbers of infected people with little education face the consequences of low public health budgets and inadequate health delivery systems. In the United Kingdom and the United States the historical coincidence of the emergence of AIDS in the gay community at a time when conservative governments were unwilling either to divert funds into research or to support anything but inexplicit, inept, and ineffective public education resulted in policies that looked, and frequently were, homophobic and designed to allow a kind of passive genocide to take place (the situation has not much improved since). In France the existence of cultural traditions that discourage networking and community organization can make dying a lonely business for those without friends or family they can look to. Everywhere there is an association of AIDS with poverty, ghettoized populations (called "risk groups"), and social stigma. Everywhere avoidance behavior on the part of the well makes people with AIDS, PWAs, feel like pariahs and, in combination with the culpabilization of AIDS (manifested by the counter-concept of "innocent victims") and the evidence of government indifference and neglect, makes the sufferer feel positioned as an expendable individual and a victim whose hasty disappearance from the scene would be widely welcomed. It is this sense of expendability and neglect that is targeted in gay writing as the product of homophobia.

But, as it has affected gay men in the West, this double calamity (medical and social) that makes the experience of AIDS so particular in the forms of its burdensomeness has had a significant historical effect: it has begun to transform the way gay politics gets done. The old (post-Stonewall) politics of liberation has taken something of a back seat to a politics of self-help, in the early AIDS years, and (especially with the appearance of ACT-UP in the late 1980s) of resistance and social intervention (see Halperin). Coming out is still important and necessary: it is the first step on which all subsequent political effectiveness is predicated. But what AIDS has demonstrated, with its *forced* comings out, is the failure of Enlightenment-style faith in the power of truth to destroy false consciousness. The new visibility that was in part forced on gay people and which has made "homosexuality" a mentionable topic in the media, for instance, and in schools, far from dissipating homophobia, seems rather to have given it new life or at least to have given it new forms and modes of action. In response to the observation that homophobia was not going away, a new style of activism thus began to emerge, a style that is more deliberately and provocatively confrontational than coming out was and displays more interest in achieving urgently needed results than in winning hearts and minds, more concern to be *heard* than to be liked or respected. "Out of the closets and into the streets" has become "We're here, we're queer. Get used to it." A style of witness that put its trust in the vulnerability of prejudice to the demonstration of truth has evolved into a more confrontational style that *assumes* stigma ("we're queer") and on occasion parades it, as the condition of having a voice in social affairs and being attended to. "Get used to it," in other words, is a direct response to the homophobic message: Go away, disappear, die off fast and without fuss.

Obviously the revolutionary implications of this change in political style and tactics should not be overstated, but it has achieved some tangible results. Physicians began to listen to what their patients had to say (in part because they were sometimes manifestly better informed than the professionals); the principles and procedures that had governed the testing of new drugs in the United States were modified in response to gay outrage and protest; and homosexuality, as I've said, previously the great unmentionable in the state ideological apparatuses (Althusser), became discussable, although not necessarily in benign terms. It still isn't okay to be gay, but for many that has ceased to be a goal (it always carried the risk of co-optation), and, if minority status in a community entails exclusion from the right to participate in what that community regards as the making of history, as I've argued (Chambers 1994), then one of the more important historical outcomes of the AIDS crisis in the West has been that the existence of gay pressure groups, and of a gay political constituency, has been acknowledged, while some of their messages have begun to register. In short, the "get used to it" part of the "we're here, we're queer" slogan has begun to happen.

AIDS witnessing texts, of which AIDS diaries form part, can be

## Dying as an Author

understood, then, as participating in the new political climate, with its stress on "audibility" (in the strong sense of "getting through") as an important supplementation of the earlier, and continuing, policy of visibility (inherent in the doctrine of coming out). It is not just that AIDS diaries and narratives are written with an expectation of publication, and indeed are often published by mainstream firms, while videos are shown on TV or (in the United States and elsewhere) may be commercially available. It's more that their mode of witness, which continues to owe something to the firsthandedness that accounts for the privileging of the eyewitness (as gay politics has traditionally relied on visibility), has been led to take account of a problematics of readability and the complexities of address—that is, the conditions of witnessing when its authority, in Benjamin's phrase, is borrowed from death. In the way that the cynical arguments of revisionist historiography (denying the reality of Nazi gas chambers on the grounds that no eyewitness account of them exists) forced the modern understanding of witnessing discourse as irreducible to a purely referential act and inevitably a practice of address, subject to the deferral of readability (Lyotard; Felman and Laub), so the writing of AIDS witness in diary form has begun to understand itself certainly as a "direct"—or, more accurately, "live"—report from the AIDS front but also as crucially conditioned, given the death of the author as both literal and theoretical fact, by a scenario of survival that entails phenomena of deferral and supplementation and hence a politics of readership that itself presupposes a rhetoric of address.

And, as in the case of the "get used to it" slogan, that rhetoric tends to be confrontational: it is the rhetoric of "face it." Obviously, the readership for a text of gay witness will always be split and diverse—other gay men, other AIDS sufferers, the homophobic and indifferent majority—and the "face it" implications of the text will have a different nuance for each constituency. But, equally obviously, the differences between such constituencies are not watertight (they overlap significantly), and only slightly less obviously they are, in addition, all subsumable under the general category I just called the homophobic and indifferent majority—a category rightly presumed homophobic because homophobia is universal in a homophobic social formation (even gay subjects are vulnerable to "internalized" homophobia) and indifferent because, in the perspective of dying authors, it consists inevitably of a population of survivors, whose interests are by definition no longer commensurate with those of the dead.

Every reader of an AIDS journal is positioned first and foremost as a survivor because it is in the context of reading that the authorial *énoncé* "I am dying" comes to be interpreted as signifying "'I' is dead." Thus, what every reader is called upon to face in the act of reading is first of all the fact of the author's death, readable in the textual uncenteredness that makes for the phenomenon of readability (an uncenteredness figured proleptically in the texts by the physical and personal disintegration they record, as also sometimes by the figure of the scattering of ashes). But every reader must also face an awareness of the responsibilities of readerly survivorhood, which are those of ensuring the survival of the text whose author is dead, and of prolonging its witness, responsibilities that, because of the inevitable difference (named by death) between readerly survivorhood and the authorial project of which the text is the only surviving evidence, are necessarily tinged with a sense of inadequacy and, almost as inevitably, with a sense of guilt. Every reading confirms, condones, and profits from the death of the author, which is why every reader, as survivor, stands accused in advance of indifference to the author's fate, through a failure to ensure the author's survival adequately, and such readerly indifference can in turn be readily identified with the homophobia that seeks to make the author a victim.

For the best survival of all would be for the author to be still alive, the impossibility of which is exactly what the fact of reading a text—realizing it as readable discourse—both entails and profits from, let's say: takes advantage of. It is the death of the author that is the condition of textual readability. Interpretation thus substitutes itself for the dead author's erstwhile control of meaning, while being unable either to restore that lost meaning (which has become irrecuperable) or (since interpretation is always specifically positioned) to endow the text with its full range of possible significations. It is neither restorative of what has been irrevocably lost nor fully able to realize the potential for signification released by that loss. In two ways, then, the reader is open to a sense of inadequacy that amounts to a form of what is called "survivor guilt." The reader's scrupulous question: Could I read this text *better?* is the moral equivalent of every survivor's anxious self-questioning: Could I have done *more* to forestall this death (to ensure the survival of the deceased)? But this question itself dis-

## Dying as an Author

places a deeper anxiety: Did I *kill* the deceased? which has its own relevance to the reading situation. For every reading displaces an author's saying (*énoncé*), and one might say "buries" it, by constructing an enunciatory situation in which authorial meaning—the *énoncé*—itself becomes a function of readerly interpretation. And, finally, in the more specific case of an author's death from AIDS, every surviving person, whether a reader or no, is required to face the question of culpability for the author's death because, on the face of it, none of us has done enough to combat the homophobic indifference that makes AIDS sufferers feel unwanted and expendable, the victim of genocide. If we are not guilty of homophobic indifference, then we are guilty of homophobic indifference to the homophobic indifference that prevails. Not surprisingly, then, the address structures through which AIDS diaries construct the figure of their reader—the reader on whose survivorhood the survival of the texts' act of witness depends—can be tinged with anger, and a barely concealed tone of accusation, that is calculated to make the actual experience of reading, of reading that address, one of anxiety, inadequacy, and guilt. This is a question I'll return to a little more fully at the end of this essay (chap. 6).

But the pattern of witness, then, as a matter of "facing it" is this. An author must face, and assume, his own death as an author, so that the surviving text, bearing witness to that death, can in turn challenge its readers with the evidence *they* must face, which is simultaneously the evidence of that death, the evidence of their own readerly responsibility for the continued bearing of witness, and the evidence of their own inadequacy fully to complete the author's interrupted task and thus to ensure the author a form of survival. There remains one further question, however. For at the origin of the chain of confrontations is another prior confrontation, out of which emerges the initial decision, on the part of a suffering human being, to die *as an author*—that is, to survive for now, and for as long as it takes to die of AIDS, so as to write and thus to borrow authority from death for purposes of witnessing.

What, then, is at stake in an author's decision, upon AIDS diagnosis, to write? Why is it triggered, on the evidence of the texts themselves, by the appearance of AIDS symptoms (in the form of an opportunistic disease) after the period of seropositivity—symptoms that not only figure the writing of the body, as I've already mentioned, and furnish the myth of the writing of AIDS but also, and perhaps first and foremost, foretell the relatively early demise of the author? Why does a professional writer who knows he is soon to die react by starting a journal? And what is the sense of the collusion with AIDS that is signaled by the decision to become the scribe of a body on which the writing that signifies death has appeared? For criticism these questions, which are "extraliterary" in the sense that the authors seem never to address them explicitly and only sometimes by implication, are nevertheless the key to the whole pattern of witnessing that emerges from the texts, as an option in favor of survival—survival in the face of death but also on the condition of death. For it seems that looking death in the face entails, in the first instance, choosing a slow, hard process of dying, as the condition of a certain survival, over an easier, and so tempting but ultimately unacceptable solution, which is that of putting an end to it all—and of forgoing, as a result, the possibility of bearing witness. It's in the form of suicide, in other words, that death must first of all be faced, and rejected, so that it can be assumed—and faced again—in the form of living with, and dying of, AIDS.

"Il me fallait vivre," says Guibert early in *La pudeur ou l'impudeur,* "avec ce sang démoli, exposé. [. . .] Est-ce que ça se voit dans les yeux? [I'd felt my blood suddenly stripped naked, laid bare. . . . Does it show in my eyes?]."[2] He thus catches the extreme sense of vulnerability to which seropositive people and PWAs alike are sensitive. Read the ads in a magazine like *POZ*—not the "viatical" ones but those inserted by pharmaceutical companies and the manufacturers of nutritional supplements—and it becomes clear that they have identified this sense of vulnerability as a major psychological response to a compromised immune system (and are proceeding to take advantage of it). It is, of course, an entirely justified response, since—as is well known—it is not the HIV virus that kills (except in relatively rare instances), but the opportunistic diseases that take advantage of the sufferer's immunological weakness. What the PWA has most to fear is infection—which is why it is both ironic and cruel that AIDS patients are treated, both medically (with all the apparatus of gowns, masks, and gloves) and socially (they are shunned), as if they were *themselves*

---

2. Cf. Guibert 1990, 14 (and trans., 6).

dangerously contagious. HIV disease is, of course, not contagious: it can be transmitted only under very specific conditions. The person who *is* vulnerable to contagion, and dangerously so, is the one in whom the appearance of AIDS symptoms (opportunistic diseases) has demonstrated the weakness of their immune system. Whence Eric Michaels's alarm and disbelief at finding himself hospitalized in an infectious diseases ward (43)—on the face of it the *last* place an AIDS patient should be put but clear enough evidence of the workings of a perverse logic that defines the PWA as a threat to other people when it is that person's life that is actually in danger. And whence, more generally, the sense of *social* vulnerability—Guibert's "Est-ce que ça se voit dans les yeux?"—that gets conjoined, as a consequence, to the PWA's sense of medical exposure.

The irrationality of treating an AIDS patient as contagious has its most likely source in the historical accident that has associated AIDS with homosexuality in Western societies and in the homophobic myth that views homosexuality itself as contagious: not just a disease, like AIDS, that can be transmitted but one you can "catch" from simple social contact with gay people. This is a myth that's rarely voiced, so fragile is its rational basis, yet, for example, in the spring of 1995 a group of gay activists (*not* PWAs) who had been invited to the White House were met at the entrance by a posse of security agents clad in gloves and masks, as if they thought that gay people could give them AIDS just by being gay. Such incidents, of which there are many, lead gay PWAs to conclude that the problem they present to society "at large" lies neither in their real (but scarcely dangerous) infectiousness nor even in the contagiousness that is ignorantly attributed to HIV disease but in the fact that, by virtue of the homosexuality of which AIDS is itself held to be an indexical sign, they are understood to be *socially contaminating agents*—a threat to some mythic "purity" from which it is felt necessary to isolate them, as Michaels was isolated in an infectious diseases ward. The phobic object, in other words, is not the AIDS-infected body per se; rather it is the figure of the homosexual, as it is constructed under the regime of compulsory heterosexuality but also as it is made visible, sometimes in a literal sense, by symptomatic AIDS: the gauntness of a wasted body, for example, or the legible marking of Kaposi's lesions. (On the persistent trope of the visibility of homosexuality, as a legible inscription on the body, see Edelman 3–23.)

The social vulnerability of the PWA is thus a vulnerability to the homophobic assessment of the patient's identity as a threat to "society" that is readable—in contradistinction to Guibert's fear that his own medical vulnerability might be legible—in the eyes of the well. After his early stay in the hospital Eric Michaels was led to write: "Mama, you wouldn't believe how people treat you there! It's not the rubber gloves, or the facemasks, or bizarre plastic wrapping on everything. It's the way people address you, by gesture, by eye, by mouth" (25/4). What is contagious, then, isn't AIDS; it's the social disease of homophobia expressed in the avoidance behavior to which the PWA is psychologically exposed: the contamination is carried "by gesture, by eye, by mouth," and its most likely outcome, when the PWA catches it, is depression and despair. For all gay men (where *gay* indicates a degree of political consciousness) are conscious of, and alert to, their vulnerability to the self-hatred that is caused—even at the best of times—by what is called "internalized homophobia." But the gay PWA is exposed to that danger in a way that is quite unusually intense and inescapable, and in his case the disease is specifically life threatening. For, given the circumstances of HIV infection and the prognosis implicit in the appearance of symptoms, internalized homophobia can easily tip the balance in the direction of despair, that "opportunistic infection of the spirit" (Monette 1990, 102) and thus immeasurably strengthen the temptation of suicide, to which the terminally ill are in any case susceptible.

I gave a brief and inadequate account of the direness of AIDS earlier in part to make it clear why suicide might not only be tempting but also appear an entirely rational response to a person recently diagnosed with AIDS. But to a gay man attempting to fight off the self-loathing induced by the status of social pariah attributed to him as an AIDS patient, suicide cannot be regarded as socially neutral and a merely personal response, however rational it may be. For it is inevitably contaminated by the homophobia, internalized or otherwise, of which it looks and feels like an outcome. Suicide is thus transformed from an understandable response to the certainty of bodily and mental suffering—that is, both a "solution" and an affirmation of personal dignity and freedom—into a hostile assault on one's own person and a form of gay bashing: the moral equivalent of murder. And it is then, in light of this inevitably homophobic valency of suicide, that the decision to write—to stay alive and to die of AIDS

## Dying as an Author

while keeping a diary of one's own death by way of performing an act of witness—becomes relevant. It is a prophylactic gesture not only in the sense, already mentioned, that it offers a means of survival beyond one's personal death but also in a more social and political sense: writing, in the context of the ever-present temptation of suicide, becomes a means of self-affirmation and self-protection against the dangerously contagious disease of homophobia, with its outcomes of self-hatred, depression, and self-destruction.

Under the circumstances of the gay male AIDS patient to choose not to kill oneself but to live—that is, to suffer the disease's indignities and to die—has, in itself already, the sense of a rejection of homophobic hatred. It signifies a choice to survive as a way of refusing to be a consenting social victim and to go quietly, in the way that, it seems evident, most of the people one meets would wish. But to write one's AIDS diary in those circumstances is, in addition, to sanction that choice of survival by ensuring that its meaning as an act of witness itself survives one's death and becomes readily and widely available (the motivation that accounts for the orientation of supposedly private diaries toward publication and readership). And it serves, finally, to underscore that meaning by making the dramatic gesture of collaborating with a loathsome disease so as to produce "the writing of AIDS," a gesture that then stands as the preferable alternative to submitting passively to the social assessment of one's worth as a pariah and a victim—an expendable individual who might just as well disappear. At the not inconsiderable cost of assuming the consequences of disease and death, a statement of social resistance is made through an affirmation of the value of surviving.

The question of suicide, and of writing—specifically of filming one's life and one's dying—as a therapeutic response to the temptation of suicide, is central in *La pudeur ou l'impudeur*, where it is explicitly thematized as we shall see (chap. 3). But even in diaries in which suicide is not an overt issue homophobia and its toxic myths are always alluded to (at least implicitly and usually explicitly) as the polarity against which the act of writing, or of filming, makes sense and becomes a form of preventive medicine, an act of decontamination that is directed both outwardly, toward the contaminating social environment, and inwardly, toward oneself. "On ne meurt que pour autrui," wrote Gilles Barbedette (82). "Jamais pour soi-même [One dies only for others. Never for oneself]"—and that is certainly true.

## Facing It

The death of the PWA, whether as an author or no, has already the sense of an act of witness and constitutes a mode of address "for others," one that the writing of a diary only amplifies and specifies. But, classically, the personal diary is the genre of introspection, self-examination, and self-knowledge, and it would be wrong to assume that, by virtue of their orientation toward publication and reading, AIDS diaries do not share in—although they perhaps transform—this traditional function. Their self-decontaminating role, with respect to a homophobic society they incriminate, should not be underestimated.

Yet it should not be taken, either, to mean that they construct their writing subject, the author, as a site of some impossible purity, unimaginable innocence, or imposing heroism. Rather, the opposite: the writing of an AIDS diary, as a gesture of self-decontamination, is in the first instance an instrument for contemplating oneself in the abjections of the body and the deficiencies of the spirit to which so dire a personal crisis, psychological as well as spiritual, reduces one, and these last inevitably include moments of internalized homophobia, self-hatred, depression, discouragement, despair. But it is precisely in this that the writing is self-decontaminating: facing down suicide, in other words, means facing up to the reasons that make it seem attractive. Authors of an AIDS diary have nothing to gain from adopting a position of anything but absolute frankness about their moments of weakness, since these are in effect the very content of their act of witness, defining the unacceptable alternative—homophobia as a socially contracted "opportunistic disease"—against which they have opted to struggle by choosing not just to die slowly and painfully but to die writing, to die as an author. And the writing of AIDS does not deny the stigma of homophobia, then, so much as it *assumes this stigma* by "choosing AIDS" while transforming its valency, making it an instrument of oppositionality.

Thus, Pascal de Duve, at one point, punningly and untranslatably writes what sounds for a distressing moment like an incredibly homophobic self-judgment: "Je meurs de mes moeurs. Je trépasse de mes passes [My sexual mores are killing me. I'm passing away because of the passes I've made.]" (33). But then he transvalues this assumed homophobia with another pun on *tant pis* (too bad): "Tant pris pour moi [So much the worse for me / So much gained by me]." "Tant pris pour moi," I think, could well be the motto of every AIDS journal, which signals the choice of survival (so much gained over death) as a sign of gay unrepentance through its embrace of a disease that, however painful and dispiriting (so much the worse for me), is deemed preferable to the judgment of a social formation that is itself lethal to gay people when it drives them to the point of suicide.

Viewed in this way, the writing of AIDS as a practice of self-decontamination, embracing AIDS in preference to the greater evil of embracing homophobia, has a structure that is not far removed from what Marie Maclean describes as "delegitimation"—that is, the symbolic assumption, and so transvaluation, by a stigmatized subject (Maclean is writing about bastards and pseudobastardy) of the stigma that brands the individual as illegitimate. "It may involve publicly laying claim to actual illegitimacy and the proud assumption of the exclusion it entails," she writes. "It may, on the other hand, be the proclamation of a symbolic illegitimacy by public rejection of the father's name, the father's values, or both" (6). AIDS diaries (like AIDS testimonial in general) look very like this second case: they constitute a "proclamation of symbolic illegitimacy" by a public assumption of the indignities of AIDS, which include the social indignities associated with homophobia as well as the always dreary and distressing business of dying in the care of modern medicine. And they make that double assumption (of AIDS and of the homophobia that accompanies it) as a repudiation of the patriarchal values entailed in the law of compulsory heterosexuality and the scapegoating of "deviant" desire.

To be sure, in the AIDS diaries I know I have not detected any examples in which delegitimation, as the "public rejection of the father's name, the father's values, or both," takes the form of an assumption of the name of the mother, as Maclean's book would suggest. But there are circumstances, surely, in which turning to writing *itself* constitutes a turning to the "the mother" and all that she, as not-the-father, can symbolize. And if that is so, and if homophobia is the pandemic disease of patriarchally ordered society, then perhaps AIDS itself, embraced as the stigmatized writing of the body of which authorial writing is a kind of transcription, is the maternal name that the writers of AIDS diaries tend to assume? In a certain situation of extremity it offers itself as the *only alternative*—not necessarily an attractive one—to the self-destruction that is a requirement of the father's law, and in that sense and to that degree it may appear seductive.

## Facing It

In the case of Pascal de Duve, as we've seen, the turn toward AIDS can reach the extreme of "Sida mon amour [AIDS my beloved]":

"Sida mon amour." Comment oser ce cri passionné? Si je n'étais que "banalement" séropositif, jamais je ne me serais permis ce qui eût été de l'indécence. [...] Mais voilà, je suis à un stade avancé de la maladie, je connais ses souffrances physiques et morales. Et c'est ainsi que la provocation devient espoir. Frères et soeurs d'infortune, ne négligez pas de puiser dans les ressources qu'offre cette maladie à votre sensibilité. Ouvrez les yeux pour vous émerveiller des grandes choses et surtout des petites, toutes celles dont ceux que la Mort ne courtise pas encore, ceux pour qui la Mort est lointaine et abstraite, ne peuvent véritablement jouir comme nous le pouvons. Sidéens de tous les pays, grisons-nous de ce privilège, pour mieux combattre nos souffrances que je ne veux nullement minimiser. (96)

["AIDS my beloved." How dare I utter this passionate cry? If I was just an "ordinary" seropositive, it would be indecent and I would never have indulged in it. . . . But there you are, I am at the advanced stage of the disease, and I know its suffering, both physical and spiritual. And that is how a provocation can become hope. Brothers and sisters in misfortune, don't neglect to draw upon the resources the disease offers your sensibility. Open your eyes to wonderment at the great things, and especially the small, all the things that those who are not yet courted by Death, those for whom Death is still distant and abstract, cannot really enjoy as we do. AIDS patients of the world, let's get intoxicated on our privilege, the better to combat our sufferings, which I do not mean to minimize.]

The element of parody in this passage (the Marx of "Workers of the world . . . ," the Baudelaire of "Enivrez-vous!") indicates a level of self-consciousness and self-irony, but the counter-mythologization is also evident. Duve has heard distressingly homophobic conversations about AIDS among his fellow passengers on the ship and has kept silent. With a certain amount of prestigious cultural reference between the lines (Baudelairean dandyism, Bataille on "sovereignty"), the stigma suffered in those homophobic conversations is converted here into a privilege (the dying author is neither an "ordinary" seropositive person nor a fortiori one of those to whom death remains distant and abstract), and that sense of privilege in turn justifies a declaration of love for AIDS that would in other circumstances be provocative but here becomes a message of hope addressed to fellow sufferers.

It is certainly true that few AIDS writers go to these lengths of lyricism. Most maintain a more confrontational stance, producing AIDS, at least nominally, as the reference of representational practices rather than as the inspirer, or even the true subject, of their writing (as in Duve's "HIV, it's pretty much you who are doing the writing here"). Others occupy the opposite end of the spectrum from Duve, reviling AIDS as a calamity, as Monette never ceases to do, or declaring it, as Michaels does, a social agent in league with the most repressive forces ("This is why I have AIDS, because it is now on the cover of *Life*, circa 1987" [29]), forces against which, as a matter of "first principles," it is necessary to struggle unremittingly. But we have seen both Monette ("AIDS has taught me precisely what I am writ in") and Michaels ("I watched these spots on my legs [. . .] taking them as some sort of morphemes") make their nod to the trope of the writing of the AIDS body, with the "delegitimatory" or decontaminatory mythologization it implies and the consequent complicity with the disease that it entails. It seems hard for the writing of antihomophic AIDS witness not to be, in some degree and in some sense, simultaneously what I have called the writing of AIDS.

As readers of AIDS diaries, then, responding to the relay structure of their mode of address by seeking to take up their interrupted practice of witness, we find ourselves faced with a text that is a kind of pharmakon, a remedy with poisonous characteristics, a poison with the capacity to cure. In the presence of texts that are complicitous with a dire disease we need to understand what motivates that complicity, so as not to fall into the complicity ourselves and so as the better to pursue the dynamics of its underlying motivation. To choose the manner of one's dying, and to construct it as a meaningful and durable statement, an act of witness that can survive one's death, is better than to choose death in preference to disease when that choice is scarcely a choice at all, because it is tantamount to submitting to a barbarous social law. Such is the option implied by the very existence of AIDS diaries, whether or not they are explicit in their reference to it, but it is an option that entails the writing of AIDS as a form of complicity with the disease. Such a pharmakon therefore implies something like cautious "dosage" on the reader's part or, if you will, a "protocol" for reading, where *protocol* has the technical sense given to it in medicine—a sense that is now sadly part of the lay lexicon among informed AIDS patients—of a set of rules that define the appropriate "delivery" of a drug.

This essay seeks to propose a protocol, in that sense, for the reading of AIDS diaries not so much as a "set of rules," perhaps, but as a way of positioning the texts such that the writing of AIDS, with the complicity and the mythologization it entails, becomes clearly understandable as an act of witness. But I realize, too, that in the age of AIDS, when treatments are experimental and the toxicity of drugs frequently unknown, protocols are mainly a matter of guesswork, and the very etymology of the term (*proton*, first; *kolla*, glue), designating the first papyrus sheet that was glued to the cylinder around which a document was rolled, perhaps suggests the idea not so much of a firm prescription as of a first stab at getting something right, subject to later elaboration and doubtless modification and correction. That, in any case, is the spirit in which I propose this essay, in the hope and expectation that it will be followed by more accurate, more appropriate, and more developed studies of an emerging genre that we have yet to learn how to read.

One thing that does seem inescapably clear, though, is that the genre forces an acknowledgment of what, no doubt, has always been obscurely understood, although I have never seen it formulated: that reading is necessarily and inescapably a form of mourning and that what it mourns is the death of the author. Furthermore, AIDS diaries require us to understand reading-as-mourning less in terms of remembrance than in terms of witnessing, and they suggest, moreover, that a form of *survival* hangs on their successful recruitment of the reader as an appropriate agent of the continued witness their own interrupted testimonial demands. They do not want the pieties of memorialization as an act of closure that makes forgetting possible; they want their own insertion in a process that is open-ended and transformative. They do not want the death of the author to deny the texts a continued historical presence and efficacy, for which the reader is made responsible.

I do not think there has been much reflection about reading in this light—that is, about reading as mourning or a fortiori about reading-as-mourning as an act of witness. We have not even begun to consider, let alone understand, the difficulties, anxieties, and perhaps impossibilities associated with such an understanding of reading, witnessing, and mourning. But the texts, one might assume, can coach us a little, since after all that is their *interest*, and, in turning to them now, I do so in some hope of deriving from a reading of their writing of AIDS a degree of instruction about the relation of reading to the responsibilities of survivorhood.

3

# Confronting It: *La pudeur ou l'impudeur* and the Phantom Image

In 1981 the first rumors of a supposed "gay cancer" began to circulate in New York. That year, in Paris, Hervé Guibert published a book about photography, his passion: the book was entitled *L'image fantôme*, which might translate either as "The Phantom Image" or "Phantom Imagery."[1] It is, idiosyncratically enough, a book about photography that contains no photographs: writing is the phantom— "un négatif de photographie" (123)—that substitutes here for images that themselves are sometimes real but equally often imaginary or fictional, unless they are photos taken but undevelopable, desired but unobtained. The photographs referred to but not presented in *L'image fantôme* thus have a quality of absent presence that signals a problematics of survival and of survival through representation: they have "died" into writing, but in the writing they survive as ghostly images. That is a reason why *La pudeur ou l'impudeur*, the video AIDS diary Guibert made in 1990–91, can be regarded, uncannily, as the necessary photographic illustration, missing from the book, of the concept of phantom imagery, an illustration that came to exist only ten years later, as a result of the epidemic whose virulence no one in 1981 could have suspected.

For, if at the start of the 1981 volume, writing is defined as the site and medium of phantom imagery, the book is so constructed that, by the end, it is photography itself that finds itself so defined. Like writing, photography is a technology of representation that produces absent presence (or present absence); it simultaneously reduces

---

1. I had written this sentence before the English translation, *Ghost Image*, appeared (see Guibert 1981). I retain *phantom*, though, because I wish to link this chapter with Emily Apter's pioneering article "Fantom Images," on *A l'ami* (*The Friend*). My *Webster's Unabridged* says that *phantom* "is also spelled *fantom.*"

its object to a state of *ghostliness* and, in so doing, ensures that the object survives the "death" (into representedness) that it undergoes as a very condition of that survival (since otherwise it would die absolutely). Thus, the final piece in the volume, entitled "L'image cancéreuse" (The Cancerous Image), tells the story of a photograph representing an attractive young man—a photograph that, or a young man who, after seven years of being admired and desired by the narrator, is attacked by "cancer": a chemical reaction produced by the glue on the photograph's back destroys the image, as cancer might eat away its human subject. "L'image était cancéreuse. Mon ami malade [The image was cancerous. My friend ill]" (167). (Thus, as in the case of "the writing of AIDS," the representation and its object are equivalent here.) But the cancer gives a new intensity to the image's eyes: "un léger accident chimique fit qu'il se mit à me regarder, à me voir alors qu'il ne m'avait jamais vu. Et je ne pus supporter ce regard qui se faisait, en même temps que la bouche, toujours plus suppliant [As a result of a slight chemical accident, he began to look at me, and to see me although he had never seen me before. I could not withstand his look, which, along with his mouth, became ever more supplicant]" (168). In an attempt to escape this confrontation with the demand of a dying subject, then, the narrator takes to wearing the photograph against his body, "comme un second frère mort attaché à moi [like a deceased second brother attached to me]," only to discover in due course that the photo has become blank, its image having been transferred to the narrator's own body, each pigment, as he puts it, finding a place in one of the pores of his skin. Far from his having eluded the image's demand, a transfer has occurred that is exact and total. "Le transfert l'avait délivré de sa maladie [The transfer had freed him of his disease]" (169).

This narrative of confrontation, transfer, and survival thus reveals itself to be an allegorical reflection on the conditions and consequences of representation, understood as a mode of *deliverance* for beings subject to death but conditioned on a rule of communicability. By inflicting death on its object, representation simultaneously forces the observer it implies to face up to the dying object and experience the intensity that emanates from it, so that, "freed" of its own disease, the object comes to survive, through a relay effect and as the result of the transfer of its image to another, who becomes its bearer. The narrative is simultaneously an allegory of reading, then, as a survivor's act that, even in attempting to shun the confrontation with an image of death in the form of representation, nevertheless ensures the survival of that image and of its dying subject—a subject whose death it is that, by the intensity it confers, makes the image a *haunting* and so, for readers, an inescapable one. Photography, like writing, is—in the words of a slightly earlier fragment of *L'image fantôme*—"au plus près de la mort [as close as one can get to death]": working in alliance with death, it imposes on the viewer a confrontation so intense as to be "indecent" (150), one that one might wish to turn away from but which proves irresistible, exerting a perverse fascination, a *hantise*.

> C. R., à qui je dis [. . .] mon désir de photographier l'acteur M. L. avec sa mère, paralysée, et sa tante, trouva ce mot pour qualifier ma demande, de "vicelarde." (150)

> [C. R., whom I told of . . . my desire to photograph the actor M. L. with his paralyzed mother and his aunt, came up with the word "kinky" to characterize my request.]

Remember that word *vicelarde* (kinky): in less slangy form (*vicieux*) it will return, ten years later, in *La pudeur ou l'impudeur,* in a context that confirms that the video is designating itself as an experiment in indecency, a representation that goes *au plus près de la mort.*

But the question there will be how to go about producing a representation that will "haunt" a television audience: how to get such an audience to *support* a ghostly representation, in the sense of tolerating its indecency but also—it is the same question—how to get it to act as the *support,* in the sense of bearer, that will ensure the relay effect by means of which the representation becomes a means of survival. And again Guibert will have recourse, as in "L'image cancéreuse," to an allegorical narrative that itself figures—as a *mise en abyme* of the text's illocutionary situation—the dynamics of survival through representation and "transfer." But he will now use his own AIDS-wasted body as a figure for the mortifying effects of representation and the ghostly image it produces and substitute the photographic representation of his own experiment with suicide, and his survival of that suicide, as the riveting equivalent of the glance of irresistible intensity that the young man of "L'image cancéreuse" acquires in his dying, a figure for the confrontation with death that the video's audience is invited to take part in by watching the video (and which it cannot escape even by attempting to elude it).

The issues that predominate in *La pudeur ou l'impudeur* are, therefore, rhetorical ones. They concern the video's address to its audience, given the indecency of a representation that gets as close as is possible—which also means as close as is permissible—to death: what are the limits of permissibility? how does the video ruse with them in order to get its audience's attention and achieve the desired effect of haunting? But they also concern, therefore, the inevitable fakery of a representation that, in figuring death, can *only* get "au plus près," as close as possible/permissible to its object, while inevitably falling short of its *actual* object, death itself, with the result that, in making its indecency *acceptable* to its audience, it permits us also, therefore, to blink at the confrontation and to elude in some sense or in some degree the gaze of death. Guibert, as an inventor of the genre of factual fiction in its autobiographical form—what Edmund White has dubbed "autofiction"—is a past master in the art of representation as an (authentic) faking of the facts, and again *L'image fantôme*, some time before *La pudeur ou l'impudeur*, had laid out the problem. In "Le faux" (The Fake) the narrator dreams that he has bought one of his favorite photographs, Alvárez-Bravo's chilling image of a young worker killed in an uprising, but discovers that Alvárez-Bravo has himself faked this representation of death, by means of a plastic mask or wrapper: it is the photograph of a living person made to look like a corpse. Although the narrator is furious at the deceit, his friend T. makes the necessary rhetorical point by reminding him of the *force* the photo had before he removed the telltale plastic cover. "Elle était parfaite, tu n'aurais jamais dû l'extraire de sa pochette de plastique [It was perfect, you should never have removed the plastic wrap]" (141). There is no witnessing that does not entail effects of mediation, some sort of "pochette de plastique." My reading of *La pudeur ou l'impudeur* will therefore necessarily be a reading of the video's rhetoric, of the plastic wrapping that makes it—with its "decent" structures of address and its representational fakery—an exemplary *representation*, "au plus près de la mort," of the dying of an author and so, for the reader (viewer), a site of confrontation with death. But it is intended as a reading also of the demand for *survival* that is made, as in "L'image cancéreuse," by the deliberately toned-down and partially faked representation of that dying. For the suicide represented in *La pudeur ou l'impudeur* is more accurately an experiment in suicide, not exactly a piece of fakery (although it may also be faked) but a sort of dicing with death that ensures the author a 50 percent chance of eluding death and so is isomorphic with representation itself, as a way of approaching death *au plus près* that is simultaneously an agent of survival. There is thus an authorial confrontation, through representation, that precedes and prepares that of the video's viewer.

I emphasize the video's rhetoricity, then, only because I wish to establish its status as an act of witness, an act inevitably bound up with the politics, the poetics, and the aesthetics of representation, because representation is a means of survival, and so of prolonged efficacy for the witnessing act. In opting to represent, I have said, and thus to perform an act of witness, the authors of AIDS diaries are implicitly choosing to die writing, as a politically desirable alternative to their simple disappearance from the scene, which could be brought about by an act of suicide. But Guibert, in *La pudeur ou l'impudeur*, in choosing to represent death in conformity with an aesthetics of photography as an art "as close as possible to death," simultaneously chooses to represent, in addition to his lengthy dying, something like his own suicide, and his survival of that suicide. By means of this bold move he is enabled to make explicit the temptation of suicide as that which would be inimical to his witnessing project by putting an end to it, while also taking suicide as a privileged object of his representation of death—that is, of the witnessing project itself, understood as an effort to force a confrontation with death on the part of its audience and so to ensure a certain "transfer," a certain survival of witnessing subjectivity. In this way he joins into a single episode what might otherwise be regarded as a double thematics, that of (the rejection of) suicide and that of (the representation of one's) dying as a mode of survival. He performs this telescoping by choosing in circular fashion to *represent* suicide itself but also by representing it as a mode of death that one experiences as a temptation, a temptation one *survives*, however, and that one survives, precisely, by representing it (with all the "fakery" representation involves).

In other authors engaged in the writing of their death, the temptation of suicide tends to remain implicit or to be barely hinted at; in my own analysis (chap. 2) the option of suicide and the option of witnessing were distinguished, for expository reasons, as an initial condition (the rejection of suicide) and a subsequent choice (the decision to write one's death) that jointly subtend the writing of AIDS diaries as acts of witness. But Guibert is explicit about the temptation of suicide, and also about the prophylactic value of the representation of one's dying as an alternative to suicide, signifying the choice of survival. In presenting them together, he also makes it necessary, then, for us to understand something my earlier analysis obscured, that the attraction of suicide is not something one puts behind one, once and for all, in order to write but a permanent temptation that continuously underlies, and so continuously valorizes, the choice to die writing. Guibert authorizes me to say that suicide is what *underwrites* the writing of AIDS in gay AIDS diaries.

Hervé Guibert was a respected but little-read writer in France until he wrote an AIDS autofiction, *A l'ami qui ne m'a pas sauvé la vie*, his first and still most famous and widely read text of AIDS witness. Invited on this occasion to appear on a much-watched literary TV show called "Apostrophes," Guibert—a good-looking but already visibly frail young man, who handled the difficult emotional and rhetorical circumstances gracefully (Boulé)—became an overnight celebrity. His book achieved large sales and was widely translated. One can readily surmise that, in making his video journal, *La pudeur ou l'impudeur*, the author of *L'image fantôme* understood both that the medium of television was open to him by virtue of his fame and that the condition of his reaching a mass audience would be rhetorical, a matter of address, and specifically of tact and discretion, if not fakery, in the representation of "indecent" subject matter. The video was made between June 1990 and March 1991 and shown on TF1 (a general audience channel) the following year, shortly after Guibert's death on December 27, 1991, with framing remarks provided by the programmers that ensured it would enjoy an authority "borrowed" from its author's demise. But it is a concern with address that is readable not only in the video's title but in a visual thematics of thinness, and of absent presence, that centers throughout on the representation of the author's own emaciated body.

Perhaps the best commentary on *La pudeur ou l'impudeur* would be a sentence from Gilles Barbedette's *Journal d'un jeune homme devenu vieux:* "La seule idée d'avoir à rendre compte, heure par heure, minute par minute, de son existence donne à celle-ci un curieux aspect fantômatique [The very idea of having to give an hour-by-hour, minute-by-minute account of one's existence is enough to make it seem oddly ghostlike] (115). In *La pudeur ou l'impudeur* it is the thinness of a body approaching "as close as possible to death" that literalizes this "aspect fantômatique," figuring AIDS as a writing of the body that makes death legible (in the visibility of bone structure beneath the skin, for example) but suggesting also, I think, not only a certain thinness of the medium of representation itself but also the careful and deliberately toned-down rhetoric that is, for an author seeking the wide audience Guibert has in mind, a necessary condition of the writing of AIDS as a discourse that speaks of death. The *pudeur* (pudicity) with which the *impudeur* (impudicity) of the video's representational gesture is effected produces, on the one hand, a certain effect of perversity (the video's kinky, "vicelard" aspect underlying the inadequacy of representation to its object, death) but, on the other—and perhaps especially for viewers/readers accustomed to the robust realism and frankness of a video diary like *Silverlake Life* or a written journal like *Unbecoming*—a sense of rhetorical restraint for which "thinness" seems an appropriate metaphor. These terms (*pudeur* and *impudeur*), literally translated as "pudicity" and "impudicity," are famously untranslatable, if only because the corresponding English words are so rare, whereas the concept of "pudeur," with its close cousin "discrétion" (discreetness), is central to middle-class social relations in France. Where *discrétion* entails respect for another's privacy, *pudeur* is a corresponding form of reticence with respect to one's own self-presentation, an unwillingness to impose on others one's emotions, one's body, one's sexuality. The "indecent," *impudique* spectacle of a body marked by disease and death thus implies as its compensatory and euphemizing rhetorical counterpart—a kind of trade-off—visible and unmistakable discursive compliance with an ethics of restraint, a tactics of understatement for which, in France, the *bienséance,* or decorum, practiced by seventeenth-century French neoclassical writers continues to provide, especially for (dominant) middle-class taste, an appropriate model.

We watch gross realities in *La pudeur ou l'impudeur* (Guibert on the toilet seat, suffering from diarrhea, for instance) and intensely charged events (his experiment with suicide). The understated rhetorical effect, the thinness of the verbal and visual writing with relation to what it represents, is at first disconcerting, like an unexpected and inappropriate perversity, and it is only with time that its efficacy becomes apparent, even to viewers of non-French culture, as images linger in the mind and indeed refuse to be forgotten, eluding one's wish to escape their impact and inviting careful and reflective interpretation. They become haunting, in other words, and the haunt is as much due to rhetorical discretion as it is to the power of images and words that are *au plus près de la mort*. The thinness of Guibert's pale and wraithlike body, making death readable as a kind of skeletal reality, is a key figure, therefore, for this strange effect of combination. But it is figured also by one of the video's two most striking narrative episodes.

Guibert is to undergo an operation, under local anesthetic, to remove "a kind of ganglion" from his neck (this description being itself a perfect example of *pudeur*, since we learn from other sources that it was a suspected lymphoma).[2] He asks his doctor about videotaping, but she is adamant: because of the draping of sheets to define the "champ opératoire" (space of operation), nothing would be visible. But Guibert politely persists: supposing he were to hold up a mirror? Her response—"Vous seriez bien vicieux [That would be kinky of you]"—is amused, affectionate, vaguely self-ironic, but dismissive. It is clear that she is voicing a social taboo: there are things one just doesn't show. Perhaps she doesn't know that in the lexicon of Parisian gay subculture *vicieux* is not necessarily a pejorative term (it frequently figures as a come-on in personal ads, for instance). In the event, although the operation *is* taped, there will be no kinky, mediating, hand-held mirror: one sees, as predicted, only Guibert's draped body and the movements of the operators. A compromise has been worked out, it seems, between *impudeur* and *pudeur*, somewhat, in this instance, to the advantage of euphemism. But it happens—this is one of those strokes of luck that can arise in live filming—that at the very site of the operation (the *champ opératoire*, if you will), an intense light source trained on the incision produces an eerie glow so bright that, in the video, one sees only the light itself, not the wound or even the hands of the surgeons. And Guibert comments in voice-over: "Cette lumière chaude, irréelle, bleue et sableuse [. . .] transforme ce qu'elle touche en source de lumière incandescente [this

---

2. The operation is described at greater length in Guibert 1992b, in which we "learn" (this text is also autofiction) not only of the suspected lymphoma but also that Guibert had resolved to commit suicide in the case of a positive biopsy.

grainy, blue, eerie, warm light . . . transforms what it touches into a source of glowing illumination]."

This transformation of the visual object into a blue glow—a sort of phantom image—can obviously stand, on the one hand, as a figure for the video's own restrained and euphemizing manner in its presentation of scenes that signify the indecency of death. But, on the other hand, it also suggests a certain calculus of enlightenment, the pursuit of thoughtfulness and intelligibility that is exemplified in the video itself by Guibert's reticent but slightly didactic voice-over commentaries, the precision of which is underscored by a perceptibly flat intonation that suggests he is reading a prepared text. Like the blue glow, they issue an invitation less to *see* graphic visual material directly than to respond reflectively and in mediated fashion to its indirectly suggested presence (an absent presence, or, in the metaphor for writing that underpins *L'image fantôme,* "un négatif de photographie"). And finally, then, the light that "transforms what it touches into a source of glowing illumination" suggests an underlying narrative scenario, the story of a transformation and perhaps, indeed, of a transcendence that might be achieved through the indirection of representation. As the indecent raw material of Guibert's bodily existence, of his dying, is transformed into a certain readability through the intervention of representational technology (it requires both the camera and the operator's light to produce the glow that becomes visible only on the tape), so a dying subject, through facing death—confronting it as close as representation will permit—might hope to outlive that experience, like the subject of the "cancerous image," through a transformation of subjectivity (from authorial to textual, say), that is, through a *becoming other,* a relay of which readability is the vehicle.

If that is so, we can extrapolate from this episode, as a *mise en abyme* of the video as a whole, that Guibert is relying heavily on the nature of his medium itself, both to signify the profound *impudeur* that the pudicity of his careful rhetoric of address simultaneously disguises and intensifies—that is, to produce for his audience the confrontation with indecency they might otherwise prefer to elude—and to produce for himself, as its initial viewer, a face-to-face with mortality that might be transformative in a personal sense ("enlightening" his understanding of death) before producing the aesthetically transformative effect of relay through which textual survival becomes possible. And, indeed, he draws attention to his medium in the final voice-over of the tape, describing video as a link between photography, writing, and film and adding, by way of explanatory comment, a somewhat sybilline statement: "L'instant présent a aussi la richesse du passé [The present instant also has the wealth of the past]." I'll return later to this statement, which I take to imply the transformative power of representational media: its suggestion is that the significance of representation is, so to speak, prospective-retrospective. One makes a video (writes a journal) now so that in the future, when the death of the author will have intervened as a theoretical and eventually also a literal event—a future that will have become a present moment in its turn—a certain richness can emerge, like an unexpected "glow" on the tape, from the initial now, which will itself have become a representation of the past. But let us begin by concentrating on the power of the media—writing, photography, film, video—to mediate confrontations with death, that is, to produce phantom images and ghostlike effects through their "reduction" of the living. For it is here that the thematics of thinness emerges as most obviously apposite, and here too that thinness shows its power to suggest another life, a transformative possibility.

From the logocentric perspective all Westerners have inherited, what the media of writing, photography, film, and video have in common is the diminishment they bring about, their representational inadequacy, with respect to living reality. Writing is an impoverished, or "thin," representation of speech and, as such, fatally removed from spontaneity, directness, and firsthandedness, the site of an absence. Photography has been considered a "spectral" medium from its invention: its subject is reduced to two-dimensional flatness and frozen into preternatural stillness. Film and video restore to the photographic image the movement of life, but it remains ghostly, however, because it is still thin; it is as if the ghost itself were walking and talking, neither fully dead nor yet quite living. All these technologies function as signifiers of death, then, because, like AIDS, they impose a "reducing plan" on the living (Michaels 98/57). Yet—since the living body dies while its representation lives on—they are also suggestive of the ways in which *technē*, by reproducing *physis* in a form that is remote from natural constraints and laws, can offer an image of survival while forcing us to confront our own death.

Their archetype, in this respect, is the reflection, or mirror image,

## Confronting It

and it is characteristic, for example, that Guibert thinks of photographing his operation in a mirror. Even more striking is the moment, early in the video, when he shows his own daily confrontation as he stands naked in front of the bathroom mirror, contemplating the death that has become visible in his wasted body: "J'ai senti venir la mort dans le miroir. [. . .] Cette confrontation de tous les matins a été une expérience fondamentale [I felt death approaching in the mirror. . . . This confrontation each morning was a primal experience]."[3] Where Guibert contemplates in the mirror his own emaciated body and his own death, the viewer contemplates, in turn, the startling thinness of another's body, replicated in the luminous, two-dimensional photographic image of the video, a kind of phantom in its own right, so that Guibert becomes the figure of a more generalized death that the video invites us to face, and to face doubly: in the image and in what the image represents. As in a mirror, we watch this frail body—often seen in movement: doing cautious calisthenics, dancing to rap without moving the feet, or just standing in the apartment, swaying rhythmically to music—living a reduced life in the flatness of its representation. Painfully gaunt, it is in other respects, however, a beautiful body: the face spiritualized by the visibility of its bone structure, a shoulder recalling the angularity of certain Picasso figures, no lesions visible. In combination with Guibert's obvious youthfulness (belied only by his cautious movements), that is a reason, perhaps, why the thinness that signifies the approach of death—the representational thinness and the thinness that is represented—comes simultaneously to suggest in addition to the approach of death a certain intensification of life, in the way that a mirror image reduces existence to flatness but can simultaneously offer an image of life transformed.

In describing Guibert's understanding of photography as a device to "absenter le réel" (make reality absent / introduce absence into reality), Buisine is right, therefore, to think of Mallarmé (39). Absence is signified in the video not only through the thematics of thinness but also, more directly, in the repeated shots that explore the layout and furnishing of the apartment, as if its occupant were elsewhere and the apartment empty, and these shots focus with particular emphasis on a writing desk strewn with books, papers, objects, and imple-

---

3. Cf. Guibert 1990, 15 (trans., 7); and 1991, 18 (trans., 6–7).

ments. This, it is easy to deduce, is a figure of the author's death in both its theoretical and its literal sense. But such absence, in the viewer's experience, is the contrary of a discursive void, because it is haunted and inhabited. It speaks only of what has disappeared, of the disappearance that has made it eloquent, as in a poem like the "sonnet en -yx" ("Ses purs ongles très haut dédiant leur onyx"): the "Master" disappears that the poem itself may speak and scintillate, more freely, more fully, more profoundly. In these moments it is, then, as if we were watching a visual image of the very authority that writing borrows from death and specifically from the death of the author: they are moments in which the attenuation, to the point of disappearance, of physical presence implies an intensified and heightened eloquence that itself owes everything to that disappearance. For an "illocutionary disappearance," in Mallarmé's famous phrase,[4] is not mute; rather, it stages death as a discursive event, productive of significance.

Thus it is that to face death in the form of the mirror image that representation makes available is also to glimpse, in the very reduction of the image, the possibility of another form of life. But it is also to understand how it is that a rhetoric of attenuation, restraint, and understatement—a discourse of thinness traversed, as it were, by a future absence—may be one of the most prodigious and powerful devices at the service of a textual afterlife.

Where the kinkiness of representational indecency, its *impudeur*, is somewhat toned down in favor of euphemism in the representation of Guibert's operation, his investment in the *vicieux* and in the quality of "fakery" that accompanies acts of representation, and in particular the representation of death, is fully manifest, however, in the second of the two major episodes in the video, in which the power of representation to approach *au plus près de la mort* without its being ever able to quite capture "death itself" is specifically thematized. Yet this episode is central not only to the video's self-reflexive interest in the conditions, effects, and limitations of representation but also, and simultaneously, to its narrative structure, as an account of the transformative outcome of the act of facing death, in the double sense of

---

4. Mallarmé's word is *élocutoire:* "L'oeuvre pure implique la disparition élocutoire du poëte, qui cède l'initiative aux mots" ("Crise de vers").

facing up to the fact of personal obliteration (and social expendability) but also of facing those things down so as, in some sense, to "survive" them. And so it finally demonstrates the sense in which this act of "facing it," as a figure for the author's option to die as a writer, functions as prophylaxis—a way of resisting the contagion of homophobia—because it is a choice of self-survival through writing (albeit at the price of the author's death) over submissive self-destruction.

The episode in question is that of Guibert's suicide, or more accurately his suicide experiment, and the key to its complex and manifold significance lies, on the one hand, in his identification of suicide as a pharmakon, that is, as he puts it in the video, a "contrepoison" (counter-poison or antidote)—a way of countering the despair induced by AIDS and its attendant social suffering, notably that produced by homophobia—and, on the other hand, in an association that remains implicit in the structure of the video but is thematically explicit in both *A l'ami* and *Le protocole compassionnel*. Through this association the availability of an experimental drug (and so access, legitimate or not, to the experiment itself) is identified repeatedly as the condition of continued survival on the part of the author and hence of his continued ability to write (i.e., to survive as a textual subject through the act of dying but of dying writing and writing one's dying). Thus, in *A l'ami* the narrator, Hervé, as a figure of the author, blackmails Dr. Chandi into fudging his test results so as to obtain AZT by threatening suicide (60, 215), and it is AZT that makes it possible for him to write the story of betrayal through which access to the vaccine that would supposedly have cured him altogether is denied (a betrayal that therefore symbolizes all the ways in which an indifferent or dismissive social order signifies to the gay PWA his expendability). Similarly, in *Le protocole compassionnel*, which covers approximately the same time period in Guibert's life as *La pudeur ou l'impudeur*, it is ddI (also referred to obliquely in the video) that gives the narrator strength to write another episode in the history of his, and the author's, dying. But in *La pudeur ou l'impudeur* the drug that, so to speak, underwrites the "writing" of the video is not an experimental antiviral but Digitaline, a proven cardiac medication that is mentioned in *Le protocole* although its name is cautiously blipped from the soundtrack of the video, presumably by TF1. As is well known, an overdose of digitalis is fatal. Digitaline, then, as a sure means of committing suicide, is the *contrepoison* to despair—a medicine of the "heart"—in the way that AZT and ddI are, for their part, medications whose toxicity is able, for a time, to hold the virus itself at bay. But, although Digitaline thus stands for suicide itself as a pharmakon, it also forms part of a paradigm of drugs that includes the antivirals, drugs that are understood as antidotes to the temptation of suicide because they offer a measure of survival and the possibility of writing.

This is because Digitaline, in *La pudeur ou l'impudeur*, permits not suicide itself but an experiment in suicide and one that is deliberately modeled on the "double blind" principle that governs clinical drug tests.[5] Consequently, what the drug comes to figure is less suicide as the choice of oblivion than the *representation* of suicide as a mode of *writing* (specifically, video writing), an "experimental suicide," if one will, that has a quite different valency, because it is a metaphor for writing, than suicide "proper." As such, it can be viewed as both a riposte to the social forces that would simply have the author disappear without trace and a bid for the textual survival of an author who dies writing, a survival the aleatory quality of which (the fact that it necessarily escapes the author's control) is signified by the implied reference to double-blind testing, in which neither the experimenters nor the subjects are aware of who is being given the actual drug and who is being given a placebo. For the point of the suicide represented in *La pudeur ou l'impudeur* is both that it is set up as an experiment (in which the experimental subject has a fifty-fifty chance of survival or death) and that it is filmed (so that the act of representation splits the author into a filmed subject exposed to death and a filming subject whose survival is assured). In two concordant ways the episode signifies both the choice of death and the option of survival. But it is quite significant, also, that in *Le protocole compassionnel* (139–40) the narrator specifies that he deliberately did not take his camera and "forgot" to take his Digitaline on the vacation to Elba that is the occasion of the suicide experiment represented in the video, a vacation during which, in *Le protocole*, the visit of Djanlouka (183–85)—who goes unmentioned in the video—reactivates a thematics of transmission and survival reminiscent of "L'image cancéreuse," the early story that can be seen as the prototype for all these narratives. Djanlouka, drawn by the desire both to see ("il voulait

---

5. My thanks to Alexandre Dauge for pointing this out to me. On the double blind, see Guibert 1990, 167–69 (trans., 142–43). For a slightly longer exploration of this question, see Chambers (1997).

tout voir [. . .] [se rincer] l'oeil du spectacle de mon squelette") and to fuck the desperately ill Hervé, has brought a condom, even though he says he wants to "risquer la mort" (risk death); it is as if he were giving himself a fifty-fifty chance in an experiment of his own. We are thus invited to read *La pudeur ou l'impudeur* and *Le protocole compassionnel*, in this respect, as complementary versions of the same facing-it or dicing-with-death narrative, with emphasis on a thematics of witnessing and transfer in one case (that of the written narrative) and in the other (that of the video) on an agonistics of facing death but in which each emphasis, in the final analysis, implies the other as its own un(der)stated corollary.

In the narrative structure of the video a long opening section precedes the suicide episode. It is ostensibly devoted to the representation of Guibert's daily life as a PWA while gradually and almost imperceptibly introducing the cognate motifs of vulnerability and despair, as if these were to be understood as a half-unconscious accompaniment to the performance of everyday tasks like taking medication and reading mail, eating, exercising, resting, or talking on the phone. Thus, we see a vulnerable-looking body subjected to diarrhea, manipulated by a physiotherapist, having blood drawn (an emaciated arm extended toward us in a gesture that seems half-supplicating), undergoing medical examination (auscultations and bizarre tests), and, of course, extended on the operating table. We watch this same thin body struggling up from bed, dressing painfully and carefully, inserting itself laboriously into a jacket; we sense its frailty and reduced ability to resist; and we begin to realize the extent to which, for Guibert, even the most elementary procedures of existence—let alone the humiliations of the disease and the encounters with medicine and its torments—have become an occasion of daily struggle. It is then that we notice the first, barely perceptible signs of his discouragement. He sits, once naked and once clothed, on the toilet seat, head in hands; he lies in bed, staring upward, hand to forehead. He has commented already on the sense of exposure his tainted blood gives him, but this sense of his vulnerability now shades, for us as for him, into an awareness of his despair.

So the realization that he is contemplating suicide, when it comes, does not come unexpectedly. The thought is specifically triggered in him, it seems (according to the logic of post hoc ergo propter hoc that is proper to the paratactic, chronicle-like form of the diary), by one particular event: the receipt of a letter. A woman Guibert knows socially (she is not otherwise identified) writes—in painfully cautious terms and long, formally constructed sentences—to apologize for a conversation in which she may not have been tactful and offers to pray for him. But (in cauda venenum) the offer is conditional, and the condition is that he renounce homosexuality, "si contraire à l'Evangile" (so contrary to the Gospel). It is soon after this homophobic attack that Guibert approaches the oracles, in the form of his two elderly aunts, Tante Suzanne and Tante Louise, both familiar to readers of Guibert from a number of other texts (beginning with *Mes parents*). Suzanne, approaching her ninety-fifth birthday, is being fed by a companion as she visibly struggles to articulate responses to Guibert's questions. Louise we have met already: an alert and hale octogenarian, she has given apposite counsel: "C'est ça qu'il faut soigner, c'est le moral [It's your morale you need to take care of]." But Guibert now comes to them both with a question: is suicide acceptable when one is suffering? Suzanne's response is clear but monosyllabic: "No," and when he pursues the issue—"Why should one continue to live?"—he gets an answer that is truly oracular because it is indecipherable. Louise, on the other hand, is more articulate: it's important for him not to give up, for the sake of those who are coming after him (she means fellow sufferers who might benefit from the medical knowledge to which his continued existence would contribute). "Would you hold it against me?" he asks. No, she would understand—but she would be desperately sorry ("désolée"), and her conclusion is firm: "Non. Ne fais pas ça. On n'a pas le droit [No. Don't do it. We have no right]." In all this there is no mention of experimentation or of filming: suicide is the choice of death in the face of life's suffering.

But it is August, and the locale now shifts to the sunshine and Mediterranean landscape of Elba (not so identified in the video), where Guibert's hesitation at first continues. He sits on the terrace, reading aloud from Walter de la Mare (credited as *Miss M.*, Editions Losfeld), a passage expressing a sense of fusion with the things of nature: "les nuages, l'eau, les insectes, les pierres [clouds, water, insects, stones]" but concluding abruptly with an unexpected judgment: "Quel nain égocentrique j'étais [What an egocentric dwarf I was]," as if to imply something like Louise's negative judgment on his desire for death. Momentarily, though, the simple hedonism of a

## Confronting It

vacationer's existence—siesta on the terrace, "a moment of pure enjoyment of life"; a juicy peach; a clean shirt donned after a cooling shower—seems to tip the balance in favor of living. Guibert contentedly hums the jaunty andantino from *Peter and the Wolf*, which has already been heard accompanying the video's "home movies" segment relating to his boyhood. In Prokofiev it is walking and continuity music; here (it becomes something like the video's leitmotiv) it signifies the will to carry on, to survive, to live. The weather turns gusty, however, and a large butterfly appears, interpreted by Guibert as a signal that Tante Suzanne has died ("Quand on me demande si je crois à la métempsychose, je dis non [When I'm asked if I believe in metempsychosis, I say I don't]"). Again diarrhea strikes, and he sits, hands covering his eyes. And we learn of the existence of the carefully hoarded antidote, the *contrepoison:* seventy drops, says Guibert, constitute a fatal dose. His face impassive, he now sits at a table, slowly and deliberately opens the vial, pours a glass of water, then another, and transfers the drug with a dropper into the right-hand glass. "Deux verres," he intones, "que je tourne, les yeux fermés [Two glasses. I twirl them, with my eyes closed]." Then, having thoroughly mixed up the two glasses, he raises one of them, toys with it thoughtfully, and finally drinks, emptying it. If it is the right-hand glass, we are watching a suicide, live.

It is not a suicide we watch, however, but an experiment in suicide, specifically modeled on the analogy of experimental drug tests and so linked to the antivirals that, to Guibert, signify the hope of survival and the possibility of writing. What is the antidote to despair? One may hesitate over the answer and seek "experimental" elucidation. Is it the "easy death" of suicide or the harder option of survival—survival in order to write and writing in order to survive? The "double-blind" structure of the episode suggests that such a suicide experiment will be a fifty-fifty proposition, but the experiment also concludes in favor of survival. After a shot of the windy terrace for continuity we see Guibert sprawled in his bedroom armchair, apparently asleep, and hear his heavy breathing, like a sigh. Then suddenly he is awake, staring. The voice-over comment, at this point, is doubly significant, emphasizing first the transformative effect of what has transpired—"Je suis sorti épuisé de cette expérience, comme modifié [I emerged exhausted from this experience/experiment, and as if modified]"—and then the role of representation in producing the transformation: "Je crois que filmer ça a changé mon rapport au suicide [I believe filming it has changed my relation to suicide]." Representation, figured as an experimental, filmed suicide, must therefore be understood as a means of facing it, of producing the mirror image in which death can be contemplated, as Guibert saw death approaching daily in his bathroom mirror but also as the viewer of *La pudeur ou l'impudeur* can read it, in turn, in the absent presence, the thinness, of the video's images. And the effect of representation, thus understood as a means of confrontation, is a change of perspective with respect to suicide. Suicide no longer beckons as an escape from despair but becomes a figure for the confrontation with death, the approach *au plus près de la mort* that makes writing, photography, film, and video the instruments of a certain survival. For, even if Guibert had died in the suicide experiment, a certain "Guibert" would have nevertheless survived as a textual subject and as a product of the filming, that is, of the death of the author captured live.

But the ability to write, that is, to capture the death of the author live, is, of course, exactly what the Guibert of *A l'ami qui ne m'a pas sauvé la vie* represented, not as suicide but as the alternative to suicide, an alternative itself dependent on access to experimental medication. The author's changed attitude to suicide, the modification of subjectivity that occurs in *La pudeur*, thus signifies the rediscovery of writing itself as both the real counter-poison to despair (figured, in this case, by Digitaline) and the agency of a certain mode of survival that itself depends on facing death. In *A l'ami* a conception of writing as the act of describing one's own dying is an implication of the novel's "dual autobiography" structure: "ce n'était pas tant l'agonie de mon ami [Muzil] que j'étais en train de décrire que l'agonie qui m'attendait, et qui serait identique" (107) ("it wasn't so much my friend's last agony I was describing as it was my own, which was waiting for me and would be exactly like his" [91]). In *La pudeur* the description of one's own dying, as a definition of writing, is what constitutes the difference between a filmed suicide experiment—corresponding structurally to the *vicieux* filming of the operation on Guibert's neck—and suicide "proper" (from which the element of "description," or representation, is absent). The modification of the author's relation to suicide that is declared to be the outcome of such an experiment can thus only refer to a confirmation of his vocation as a writer, threatened by the temptation of suicide proper—the vocation to die writing and to write one's dying. And it is to this transformation of the author into a subject of writing, a transformation of subjectivity that simultaneously amounts to a modified relation to death itself, that the final minutes of the video are devoted.

Guibert first goes to the sea and bathes, as if in celebration of a new self, emerging from the water to be carried to the beach in the arms of a companion, whose appearance in the video (not counting doctors' visits, interviews with the aunts, the occasional phone call, and a successful author's voluminous mail) is the first real sign of a break in the relentless solitude of Guibert's existence, the sense of *having to make it on one's own* that has been conveyed throughout, as the essence of what it means to live with AIDS. This brief allusion to the friends who figure prominently in Guibert's written texts but are virtually absent from the video perhaps signifies the return of a sense of community that might be connected with renewed faith in writing (which implies the address structure of witnessing as an appeal to readers). In any case, back in Paris, life appears to resume much as before: another doctor's visit, another conversation with the oracular Tante Suzanne: "C'est dur d'être si vieux? [Is it tough to be so old?]." "Oh, yes." "What gift would you like for your ninety-fifth birthday?" "To survive a bit longer [De vivre encore un peu]." But thus the motif of the will to survive is recalled, and Guibert's own overcoming of the threat of death is suggested now in the passage he reads from a war novel, credited as *Moreau de Klabund* (Editions Le Temps Qu'il Fait-Cognac). "Moreau regardait maintenant la mort en face sans ciller," it begins ("Moreau could now look death in the face unblinkingly"), and it goes on to explain that Moreau is no longer troubled by the deaths of his military comrades, which have come to seem normal, while he is moved instead—a bit like the moment on Elba authorized by Walter de la Mare, when Guibert took pleasure in and identified with the simplest manifestations of nature—by a dead hedgehog, which he buries with some ceremony and supplies with an epitaph: "Ci-gît un hérisson [Here lies a hedgehog]." Looking death in the face does not entail insensitivity or callousness, then, although it makes death seem normal, but neither does it entail the judgment of egocentricity (as suicide did). Rather, one emerges into a new sense of survival, which produces a certain objectivity and a sort of equanimity, together with a sense of the oneness of nature.

A similar detachment from the mortal affairs of humans is evident in the following scene, the only one in which, by contrast with his earlier signs of despair, we see an amused Guibert, who even demonstrates a capacity for laughter. He is in bed, describing to a friend the scene at the lawyer's office, Tante Suzanne having died, when the family, which has gathered rapaciously from all over France to hear the will, learns that she has left all her money for cancer research. (He adds, more thoughtfully: "I saw a face of my father I didn't know at all.") Suzanne's message from the grave (recall the butterfly) reads like a message of affection and solidarity with Guibert, at the same time as it comments ironically, from the perspective of death, on the pettiness of mortal preoccupations such as money. And the final images of the video, each of them a key moment referring back to earlier images and resituating their significance, now articulate his attainment of a certain resolve, a certain faith in writing, and a certain understanding of textual survival that relativize, if they don't assuage, the pain of the author's own approaching death.

Through a doorway we see obliquely into the bedroom. An alarm goes off; a light is turned on. Pause. Two spindly legs thrash the air, and Guibert comes into view, now sitting upright on the edge of the bed. He sits, looking away from the camera, then turns his head to look upward in the other direction. The suggestion is still one of struggle but not now of despair (head in hands): instead, a certain firmness of resolution, the desire to battle on, is conveyed. And so, in a second sequence, we see him at his desk, word processing—an image that countermands an earlier image of the empty desk, strewn only with books and writing materials, and more particularly one (with the lamp alternately turned on and turned off) that signified Guibert's hesitation over suicide (to write or not to write). Correlatively, the final image of the video will be of the desk again but with Guibert absent once more, in an unmistakable figuration of the author's death. This image of absence is now so framed, however, that we see it as if presided over by an almost anthropomorphically shaped, if skeletal, lamp, one that was associated, in a carefully composed earlier image of Guibert exercising, with his own thin body. This lamp is thus something like a phantom image of the absent author, whose spectral survival and absent presence in his writing it thus signifies, even as it serves, more distantly, as a reminder of the incandescent glow that transformed the surgical operation, as a result of its representation, into a source of light.

Mallarmé is certainly in the intertext here:

Ses purs ongles très haut dédiant leur onyx,
L'Angoisse, ce minuit, soutient, lampadophore,
Maint rêve vespéral . . .

[Dedicating on high the onyx of her nails
Anguish, this midnight—a lamp-bearer—supports
Many a vesperal dream . . .]

But in the soundtrack it is Prokofiev we hear, the andantino again. For it is clear now that, Peter having faced down the Wolf, the music can continue.

Guibert has freely admitted, in *A l'ami* (159 [135]), to a lifelong fascination with death; and it seems that the "feeling" of death, as he calls it—"la peur et la convoitise" (fear and desire)—impregnates his writing from the start. Before they knew themselves to be infected, he and his friend Jules regarded AIDS as a "wondrous" disease, therefore—"une maladie merveilleuse" (*A l'ami* 192)—because it permits life, so to speak, to observe itself dying, while concomitantly death gains access to, and comes to inhabit, the world of the living. "C'était une maladie qui donnait le temps de mourir, et qui donnait à la mort le temps de vivre, le temps de découvrir le temps et de découvrir enfin la vie [It was a disease that gave one time to die, and gave death time to live, time to discover time and in the end to discover life]" (164; trans. modified). And the writing of AIDS, in Guibert, as an intensification and specification of his long-term association of writing with death, in which textual writing models itself, as phantom imagery, on the writing of a body reduced to spectral thinness, functions in turn like AIDS itself. It brings life as close as it can come to death (by giving one time to die) while simultaneously making death an inescapable presence in life (by giving death time to live), the first experience, that of drawing closer to death, being more particularly that of the author as he writes his dying, while the second, that of receiving death as a visitation in life, is more characteristic of a reader or viewer in the presence of a writer's text (a text whose significance derives from the death that is its readable subject, both in the sense that it is about dying and in the sense that death is therefore what speaks in and through it).

But by the same token AIDS does introduce a new moment into Guibert's long-term fascination with death. For his writerly complicity with a disease that makes it possible to write one's dying, and thus to make death readable, also implies a scenario of survival, the kind of scenario to which he refers in *Le protocole compassionnel:* "Je suis dans une zone de menace où je voudrais me donner l'illusion de la survie, et de la vie éternelle. Oui, [. . .] j'ai horriblement envie de vivre [I'm in a constantly threatened zone in which I would rather allow myself the illusion of survival, of eternal life. Yes, . . . I have a horrible yearning to go on living]" (143). What I want to suggest, then, is that it is the grafting onto the writing of death of various scenarios of survival, whose prototype, I have suggested, is the story of "L'image cancéreuse" in *L'image fantôme,* that most strikingly characterizes the writing of AIDS in Guibert's hands, whether it be that of the prose trilogy (*A l'ami, Le protocole, L'homme au chapeau rouge*) or that of the video diary, *La pudeur ou l'impudeur.* And what this scenario turns on, in the video, is a dynamic of confrontation that is structured precisely as an author's experience (bringing life as close as possible to death) and a reader's or viewer's experience (bringing death within the purview of life) but is in each case bound up with the power of technologies of representation. In choosing to represent his own dying (filming a biopsy operation or a suicide experiment, for example), the author is led first of all to face his own death, like Guibert in the bathroom mirror. Thus, the only close-up shot of a face in the whole video captures the intensity of Guibert's looking while he watches on the monitor the images of his operation and observes the eerie blue glow that emanates from them. But the existence of a representation of the author's dying, together with the split authorial subjectivity such a representation implies (a represented subject who dies but a representing subject, or more accurately a subject of representation, that has a chance to survive) is, in turn, the condition of a viewer's ability to confront death in the author's text and, consequently, of the survival of the subject of representation that exists only as the object of reading. The suicide experiment in *La pudeur ou l'impudeur,* under-

## Confronting It

stood (as I've proposed) as an allegory of representation, appears to estimate the chances of such a survival through representation at 50 percent.

For the responsibility, ultimately, is out of the hands of the author who is to die, since it depends on the indispensable cooperation of a viewer with the sensitivity to read the writing of death, the phantom images that the text itself can only propose. The status of the reader or viewer as a survivor of the author's death—the reader's survivorhood, that is—does not necessarily guarantee the survival the text demands. Rather, the whole problem lies in the difference between those two words. How can the reader's survivorhood be parlayed into textual survival? That problem underlies the appeal for reading that is implicit in the final voice-over commentary of the video, accompanying the spectral images of the empty desk and the lighted lamp. Ostensibly, the commentary is a meditation on the powers of representation:

> Il faut avoir déjà vécu les choses une première fois avant de pouvoir les filmer en vidéo. Sinon, on ne les comprend pas, on ne les vit pas: la vidéo absorbe tout de suite, et bêtement, cette vie pas vécue. Elle peut aussi faire le lien entre photo, écriture et cinéma. Avec la vidéo, on s'approche d'un autre instant, d'un instant nouveau, avec comme en superposition, dans un fondu-enchaîné purement mental, le souvenir du premier instant. Alors, l'instant présent a aussi la richesse du passé.
>
> [One needs to have already lived life in order to be able to video it. Otherwise it can't be grasped, it can't be lived: the video absorbs this unlived life immediately and unintelligibly (banally). It can also link photography, writing and film. With video, you can approach another instant, a new instant, which is superimposed as in a purely mental dissolve shot, on the memory of the original instant. Then the present instant also has the wealth of the past.]

What is said here seems to mean that the power of video (of representation) depends on its ability to introduce deferral, and hence a certain distance, into the unintelligible spontaneity of "unrepresented" living. Such deferral, to extrapolate, is at one and the same time the discursive sign of death and a necessary condition of signification ("life" must be mediated in order to be what we call life). But it implies also, in Guibert's analysis, a second deferral within the first, a two-stage operation that I've already called prospective-retrospective and which is where the appeal to reading comes in. For the living must become the live in order to achieve significance, intelligibility, and life—that is the prospective stage. But the (potential) readability of this live representation, if it is to produce the *fondu-enchaîné* effect of survival, by which a present moment can acquire, across time, "the wealth of the past," must in turn be realized. That is, it must be subject to an act of reading, which constitutes the stage of retrospective interpretation. Thus, the whole analysis culminates in an implicit appeal for the video to be read.

What gives this appeal its urgency, though, is the further implication that there is an intervening moment that differentiates the prospective stage of representation—a stage subject to authorial control but in which the living, in order to become (potentially) significant, is reduced to the live and thus undergoes a form of death—from the retrospective stage of interpretive realization: the enrichment that realizes the potential inherent in the live, a stage that is beyond the author's control because it implies the involvement of an agent of reading. This intervening moment can be pinpointed as the moment of the author's death. But it is therefore a moment beyond the reach of discourse, a moment that (unlike the author's dying) cannot be represented but, equally (unlike the text that survives the author's death), cannot be interpreted. There is only, on either side of the prospective-retrospective process that is structured by the writing-reading relation, a double and complementary experience not of death "itself" but of approach and confrontation. There is only the *au plus près de la mort* experience of representation, or of reading, as facing it, one that gets as close as possible to, but is not identical with, the unrepresentable, unsayable, unreadable reality. Thus, an author must confront death in the process of dying so that a reader, defined by the status of survivorhood, can in turn confront death in the textual representation of the author's dying and so produce a kind of survival that links the moments of before and after—technically, the text as *énoncé* and the text as *énonciation*—across the chasm of death "itself." But death itself divides them, defines an unbridgeable *difference* (the difference of deferral) between author and reader, and thus inevitably questions the quality of textual survival. The reader is asked to countermand the effect of something that is insurmountable: the interruption that is death.

I read the phrase "la richesse du passé," and the idea of the wealth of the past enriching the present instant of reading, as an enticement to a certain readership that we must understand, in the first instance, as a TV audience unlikely to be predisposed to welcome the *impudeur* inherent in the writing of AIDS, let alone the task of compensating for the effects of death. It is a comfortable idea and one that corresponds to traditional understandings of reading as the enrichment of reader by text and/or text by reader. There is something familiar and middle-class about it. Other texts, such as *Silverlake Life* and *Unbecoming*, to which I am about to turn, position the reader as survivor less comfortably, and indeed in considerably bleaker terms, as the site not of an enrichment but of mourning. What remains fundamental in Guibert's video, though, and gives it, along with the corpus of texts in which it is embedded, a primary place in my investigation of the relation of reading to the responsibilities of survivorhood is that—prior to the question of the nature and quality of readerly response—its understanding of writing as phantom imagery, and of the haunting of a reader to which such writing therefore gives rise, implies the very *necessity* of responsive reading. According to traditional understandings of the spectral, a ghostly visitation is one that, by virtue of the uncanny ability it demonstrates to cross the supposedly absolute boundaries assigned to death and to life, cannot be ignored. It makes not just a request of the living, whom it positions as survivors, but a demand. It requires of them that they *attend*.

The rhetoric of discretion, the spectral imagery, the thematics of thinness in Guibert—his haunted writing and his poetics of haunting—thus link with something fundamental about witnessing discourse in general and the witnessing of AIDS in particular, in that they define the responsibilities of survivorhood in terms of a requirement of response. But, when all is said and done, the response required by a haunt is less likely to imply enrichment than to entail the duties of mourning, and the question of the readerly attention that is due to phantom imagery tends to resolve, therefore, even in Guibert, into a question concerning the nature of mourning and the sense in which a reader might be said to be a mourner. A spectral visitation is traditionally held to convey a demand that the soul of the departed be permitted to rest. But how does that square with the appeal for survival—that is, for a lengthy discursive afterlife—that, as we've seen, a text, as the site of its author's death, makes on the reader? Can mourning, and can reading as mourning, ever be brought to resolution? Or is it, rather, that mourning and reading are necessarily processes both terminable and interminable, processes that defy resolution, therefore, given the contradictory desire that seems inherent in both: to lay the dead to rest but also to ensure their endless survival? It is questions such as these that, as I've said, one may expect to resurface as my investigation proceeds; they hover, wordlessly in one case but almost explicitly in the other, at the horizon of the scenarios of confrontation and survival that are readable in both *Silverlake Life* and *Unbecoming*. But they are already implicit in Guibert's definition of writing, and of the writing of AIDS, as phantom image.

# 4

## An Education in Seeing: *Silverlake Life*

In *Silverlake Life: The View from Here* (1993) the videomaker Tom Joslin—with technical assistance from a number of friends (including his lover, Mark Massi)—made a remarkable video record, in diary form, of his own dying and death from AIDS. Completed by Peter Friedman, the video is nevertheless a remarkable instance of the autobiographical genre: the role played by Mark Massi, who is also ill, makes it something of a "dual autobiography," while the technical characteristics of the camera make it possible to narrate not only the author's dying and death but also the forms of his postmortem survival as well as to explore the relation of (Mark's) survivorhood to (Tom's) survival in a way that captures something of the problematics on which I focus in this essay.

*Silverlake Life* thus takes a narrative step beyond *La pudeur ou l'impudeur*, in that suicide is not really an issue here, much less a temptation, so central to the video is its thematics of premortem living on and posthumous survival. But it also represents a rhetorical shift in that the medium is understood less as the producer of phantom imagery than as a means of making visible that which people might prefer not to see, a device for showing. Gone, then, is Guibert's discretion and sense of decorum with respect to the viewer, and the rhetoric is that of a stark representation of a grim reality, so that the thematics of confrontation, and even of visitation, have a different valency. They have to do now with an emphasis, on the one hand, on a politics of visibility that derives explicitly from the liberationist era of coming out and with an interest, on the other, in the semiotics of "the writing of AIDS," a certain power of the sign for which the visible markings of Kaposi's sarcoma are taken to be paradigmatic.

*Silverlake Life*, in short, requires of its viewer a certain courage, to match that shown by its subject(s) and maker(s): we are challenged to *see* the facts of life with AIDS, and of death from AIDS, which the video *shows* as frankly as it knows how, confronting the way things are—the "view from here"—with a sort of unblinking matter-of-factness that calls on the audience to face up to the same bitter perspective with equal lucidity. At the same time, though, the Silverlake house—by contrast in particular with Guibert's near-empty apartment, haunted by its wraithlike occupant—seems *full* almost to the point of over-occupancy: cluttered with objects, furniture, and equipment, with a visiting hummingbird and a resident cat, and, more especially as Tom's death draws close, frequently visited by friends and even family. In the manner of its making as well as in its subject matter it is a video about community, not solitude (see Seckinger and Jakobsen 1997). It is a given, part of the view from here, that community is an appropriate and strengthening response to suffering and death, and the video thus issues an invitation to its viewers to join its community, as it were, subject only to the qualification of being able to see with honesty what we are being shown with clearsighted courage and integrity.

But such an ability cannot, of itself, be taken for granted, and for that reason hypocrisy and homophobia, because as forms of denial they entail the inability to see, become the video's principal rhetorical targets. Its aim is the conversion of the phobic *look* (simultaneously homophobic and AIDS-phobic) into an ability to see, the ability to face it, because it is the inability to see that disrupts the formation of a community to which—because community is the appropriate response to the depredations of disease and the fact of death—the values of survival are attached. The rhetorical practice of showing is the video's means to that end, and what it proposes, then, is an education in seeing that targets overt homophobia but also the less easily recognized and acknowledged homophobes that sleep within us all.

Such a confrontational rhetoric of showing situates *Silverlake Life* not only in a different cultural context but also, as I've mentioned, in a different political history from *La pudeur ou l'impudeur*. Its requirement of seeing derives from the truth-telling ethics and the politics of visibility in which post-Stonewall liberationism was grounded, and the form of homophobia it targets is the homophobia of denial—the refusal to acknowledge what is the case, encapsulated these days in the U.S. military's policy of "don't ask, don't tell," that seems so characteristic of, although certainly not specific to, middle-class America and has historically determined so much public policy and so many media representations of AIDS in addition to the social institution of the closet. The passing years having demonstrated the resiliency of homophobic denial in the presence of truth-telling gestures and exasperation having mounted in consequence, the old liberationist rhetoric of standing up to be counted has clearly become more confrontational in the age of AIDS. But the need to bear witness has become more urgent also as homophobic denial took on genocidal characteristics in alliance with the lethal epidemic, and witnessing discourse correspondingly learned to borrow its authority from death. *Silverlake* obligingly permits us to measure these continuities and differences by quoting its own political past in the form of an extract from the coming-out video *Autobiography of a Close Friend*—an eerily predictive, if slightly closety, title—that Tom Joslin and Mark Massi made in collaboration back in the era of bell-bottoms and long hair.

This extract includes interviews with Tom's parents: a smiling but evasive Mary Joslin ("I don't know how frank I should be about this") and a downright uncomfortable Charlie, who declares: "I don't think you ought to advertise [homosexuality]. . . . It doesn't seem quite normal. To us. The normal people." Thus, the family (as opposed to community) is identified as the very site of homophobic denial, which in *Silverlake* will therefore become associated with the frosty winter landscape of New Hampshire, by contrast with Southern California's sunshine, flowers, and sparkling lake. How to resist the influence of family? In *Autobiography* the antidote to familial hypocrisy and the imposed secrecy of the closet ("you learn not to tell people, and to hide things") was truth-telling: "I'm tired of lying, so I make this film," said Tom, and, accordingly, Mark climbs to a snowy rooftop, from which he reads a liberationist text in a loud, clear voice ("Blatant is beautiful"). The alternative, as his flat comment makes clear when he is asked his opinion of Mary and Charlie's discomfort with him and the role he plays in their son's life, is the suicidal despair to which homophobia reduces so many gay men. In *A l'ami qui ne m'a pas sauvé la vie* Guibert records his desire "de mourir à l'abri du regard de mes parents" (16) ("to avoid dying in the spotlight of the parental eye" [8]), and it is not impossible that Guibert's attraction to suicide is related to his desire to escape dying under the gaze of the "parental eye." But in *Silverlake Life* the filming of Tom's

*Facing It*

dying and death can be regarded both as a continued option in favor of public visibility (in lieu of a quiet suicide, for example) and as symbolically dedicated to the eyes of the parents in New Hampshire, with the goal, or perhaps some less conscious motivation, of bringing them, through an education in seeing, into closer relation with the Californian community.

When *Autobiography* was shown on PBS, we learn in *Silverlake,* there was "consternation" in the family (presumably at the public airing of the secret). Consternation but also, apparently, little change: in *Silverlake Life* the parents are still in denial, although now it is denial of the disease as well as of homosexuality: "It's, like, 'it doesn't exist,'" comments Tom's sister-in-law, discussing the unwillingness of Mary and especially of Charlie to fly to California when Tom first became dangerously ill. Mark, too, is still a suspect figure in the parents' eyes. Whatever the satisfactions of truth-telling from the rooftop and whatever the consternation it may cause, nothing essential seems to have come out of it. *Silverlake,* by contrast, records an at least partial conversion on the parents' part: after Tom's death Mark will be "adopted," especially by Mary, as her son, an adoption that thus figures a certain survival of Tom himself, redivivus in the person of Mark, who is now cherished by Mary as Tom had been. Mark thus symbolically enters the Joslin family, it is true, but, equally, both parents have been induced to come to California, and we see Mary in particular interacting there with the friends of Tom and Mark as well as with Mark. The "adoption" has been a two-way process.

But the irony, as Mark points out, is that "Tom had to die for her to see how much I really did love him": if Mark's tending of Tom has functioned as an effective act of witness and made an impact on the parental homophobia, so that Mary now *sees* what she was unable and unwilling to acknowledge before (the reality of gay love), his witnessing has had to borrow its authority from death—the death of Tom—in a way and in a sense that were inapplicable in the days of truth-telling and coming out. Showing, as the later video now understands it, draws its rhetorical power, the power to convert the phobic look, less from a simple faith in visibility—the visibility of coming out and of "Blatant is beautiful"—than from a pedagogy that entails a longer and more difficult process: that of learning to confront, and to see, disease, suffering, and death.

An Education in Seeing

These lessons—the authority of death and the efficacy of a pedagogy of showing—will be made explicit by two of the three speakers at Tom's memorial service. Whitey, his elder brother, recalls Tom's "dream" of making *Silverlake Life* and mentions a recent conversation he has had with Mark, as Tom lay dying, "about destiny." "Perhaps it was his destiny to die so that *Silverlake Life* could have its full impact." Whitey is not a literary critic—he is in the air force—so his statement is a remarkable one, not only because it recognizes the rhetorical authority of death but also because his concept of destiny acknowledges a certain survival of the autobiographical subject, beyond his death, in the reception (the "impact") of his text. This differs from the more "personal" survival of Tom, replaced by Mark in Mary's affection, because it recognizes, at least implicitly, the significance of a project of witnessing and the power of technologies of representation, in this case the camera, to extend the life of the subject they represent, albeit on the ironic condition, yet again, that such an afterlife presupposes the death of the subject (that being what Whitey can be taken specifically to mean by destiny). His comment thus provides a context in which to understand the video's persistent foregrounding of video technology and the practicalities of its own making: cameras, tapes, monitors, the paraphernalia, but also the process, of filming and viewing, which frequently occupies the video makers' attention without their feeling the need, on their own part, to engage in extended theoretical discussion of them. (There is, for example, a scene in which Tom and Mark lie on the bed, filmed as they scrutinize themselves and each other in the video monitor, and another in which Tom gives us a guided tour of the equipment that fills his bedroom and so, later, will intrude on the very scene of his death.) These are the instruments through which the death of the subject can have "impact" and the subject enjoy, therefore, a "destiny."

But they are also vehicles of showing, and so of the video's confrontational tactics with respect to its audience and the education in seeing that it seeks to provide. This audience, as it is figured by Tom's parents, is assumed to be homophobic and a site of denial, the unwillingness to see. But at the service a young man, who is not identified, draws attention both to the pedagogical dimension of showing and to the range of its address. He speaks of his friendship with Tom and Mark and of the particular quality of their relation to him: they *showed* him gay life; they *showed* him their life as a couple. As professional video makers, showing is of course their business. But this is about something different: it is about the courage to eschew the privileges of privacy in the interests of cultural reproduction, the education of those, such as gay men, who, as subcultural subjects, are at best unacknowledged and at worse stigmatized in the official sites (schools, churches, the media) in which "mainstream" cultural identities are fostered (Chambers 1994).

Because of its role in maintaining the continuity of subcultural life, the teacherly role the young man refers to is particularly prized in the gay male community, and thus one can see the sense in which *Silverlake Life*'s educational project is finally a double one: not only to show those who, homophobically, do not wish to see what it is that they should learn to face but also—beyond teaching gay life and gay coupledom—to teach those who in the age of AIDS may be called upon most directly to bear witness, as Tom and Mark do, to what is at stake in choosing to face the reality of death from AIDS by recording it. There is, in short, a lesson in courage to be given as well as a project of showing to be accomplished, and it is perhaps the entanglement of the two—the courage is that of showing, frankly and honestly, what is entailed in the encounter with death, the showing of that encounter has as its object to induce such courage in others—that best characterizes the video as an education in seeing.

It might be fair to say, though, that as educators Tom and Mark collaborate by fulfilling somewhat different roles: broadly speaking, it is Mark who figures the courage entailed in showing, while Tom teaches, by example, the courage required to face death. There is a moment in Paul Rudnick's comedy *Jeffrey* (49) when the eponymous hero is set upon by gay-bashing thugs. Jeffrey claims to be armed:

*Jeffrey:* You have weapons. So do I.
*Thug #1:* I got a knife. What do you got?
*Jeffrey:* Irony. Adjectives. Eyebrows.

These, in the face of even more extreme duress, could be said to be Tom's weapons also: it is not simply that he permits the most intimate details of his dying to be captured live on tape but that he demonstrates at death's approach a form of philosophical wisdom, a stoic courage, that has a distinctly queenly twist. His is a kind of lucid realism, one conscious of the temptations of denial and the threat of despair, tempered and humanized, however, by a wry irony that indicates at once a refusal to be defeated—the rejection of victimhood—and an avoidance of pathos.

He makes a point, for example, of repeating for our benefit a doctor's graphic description of the effects of cryptococcus meningitis (this is his realism), adding only (this is the spirit of resistance), with an appropriate *moue*, "Lovely!" A walk in the Huntington Gardens, where each bench proposes a dilemma (whether to rest or to take the risk of pushing on to the next one), becomes, mock-heroically, the occasion for "a brave effort of physical dynamism." A playful metaphor (the invalid venturing onto the terrace is enjoying a Mediterranean tour) turns grim (the voyage will be short) and is "lightly" dismissed: "That's life!" I do not want to suggest that Tom is glib. He is emotionally frank (about his love for Mark, about his anger, his anxieties, his depression); he is philosophically thoughtful about the approach of death ("There's a certain amount of desperation in relation to [. . .] videotaping as compared to other parts of life") and about his own increasing detachment—first as a gay man, then as a PWA, now as "a living dead"—from existence and its absurdities. But lucidity and frankness never spill over into self-pity. When he reports that his physician has advised him to look for a hospice, knowing that this implies an average life expectancy of two months, it was, he says with characteristic understatement, "very startling to hear [. . .] and greeted with very mixed feelings," adding only, "A real bombshell." The tone is close to matter-of-fact, and the slight euphemisms ("startling," "mixed feelings") acknowledge the emotional impact honestly while expecting not pity but empathy. And, as he becomes weaker and can scarcely talk, he will continue to demonstrate the same stoic humor, waving at the camera like the queen of England at one moment and acknowledging at another that he feels "not chipper."

Whereas Tom sets an example in his way of facing death, then, showing in a more confrontational and antihomophobic sense is more specifically Mark's domain. This is in large part by virtue of the accidental fact that, although both lovers have visible KS lesions (and increasingly so as time passes), Mark from the outset is the more marked of the two, on face, limbs, and back. Kaposi's sarcoma, to which gay male AIDS patients are thought to be particularly prone, enjoys special status in the lineup of opportunistic diseases because the visibility of the lesions makes them legible as an indicator (and so easily interpretable, to the homophobic imagination, as stigma) not solely of AIDS but also of homosexuality: it is used to this effect, for example, in the Tom Hanks vehicle, Jonathan Demme's film *Philadelphia*. KS thus easily becomes the site of a certain anxiety about visibility, of which the terms are, on the one hand, ostentation (a version of "flaunting it") and, on the other, denial. For the lesions, of course, *can* be cosmetically concealed, but to a politically conscious gay man such a practice is inevitably dubious, because it smacks of the closet. It is symptomatic, therefore, that in *Silverlake* we see Tom applying cosmetic to his face in the plane that is taking him and Mark back to New Hampshire for a family Christmas—an event that will prove to be a nightmare of forced gaiety and uncomfortable denial, so that Tom will return, as he says, "sick, exhausted and unhappy with my family." His enforced complicity with parental denial—as much a denial of homosexuality as of AIDS—has been experienced, in short, as a denial of self and in that sense a step toward death. Toward a death imposed by the homophobic unwillingness to see, as opposed to death faced clear-sightedly and converted, as in the video, into an occasion of witness and the object of an education in seeing.

In California, therefore, and by contrast, both lovers are matter-of-fact and very open about showing their lesions. The episode in which they watch themselves on the monitor, photographed in profile, ends with Tom's discovery of a new lesion on Mark's left eyelid (Mark rejoices wryly, and as it turns out erroneously, that he is the one who has been chosen for the torment of having "a little lead shield" in his eyelid). Mark is examined by an herbalist, his back a mass of lesions; later he undergoes strontium-90 treatment (commenting that it was once something one feared in milk); toward the end of the video he returns to Dr. Matt, the lesions still more numerous and prominent; in each case he discusses them objectively and dispassionately, while the camera records the visual evidence. Similarly, as Tom lies near death, Mark brings the camera in for a close look at the lesion that has recently appeared on Tom's eyelid: "He says it hurts him now." KS, as the form taken here by the writing of AIDS, is thus at the center of the video's strategy of showing.

But the anxiety associated with visibility, and particularly with being looked at—when the look signals discomfort, homophobia, the

An Education in Seeing

unwillingness to see—surfaces in a scene that situates the video's practice of showing, quite specifically, as an antihomophobic gesture. Tom, at this juncture, is still able to get out, and the two are swimming in a private pool lent them by an understanding neighbor, who has nevertheless specified that Mark must wear a shirt in the pool so as not to "freak people out." In the absence of other observers (except the camera) they enjoy the water, Mark with his torso uncovered. The neighbor appears: nothing is really said (they explain, however, that they are taking advantage of the fact that no one is about), but when she leaves Mark withdraws into a covered space—referred to as a "cubby hole" (as if it were a variant of the closet)—at the end of the pool. As he does so, he pauses, however, to display his back to the camera. "Flashing me your KS?" asks Tom. "Yes. I was being political," is Mark's response. The allegory of the video's own confrontational rhetoric could not be more explicit.

But the episode also explores the kind of victory over one's own complicity in social cover-up that is entailed in "flashing one's KS." Early in the video Mark has discussed the question of telling people he has AIDS; the problem, he says, is that "they start to look at you that way. [. . .] You can't live like that. To have people looking at you like that is really uncomfortable." Now he explains his discomfort at acquiescing in the neighbor's stipulation that he cover his body. "I do that, but it feeds into that bad part of me that I don't. . . .You know, of being self-conscious and disliking my body and what-not. [. . .] I don't want to upset people, having to look at ugly me." Mark's vulnerability as he speaks is visible in his posture: crouching self-protectively, his head hunched against his shoulder. It is both a vulnerability to being looked at "that way" and a susceptibility to homophobic cover-up and self-hatred ("ugly me" as self-assessment), the urge to retreat into the closet.

Flashing his KS, and by extension Mark's participation in the whole enterprise of Tom's video—and so, ultimately, the video itself, as it is figured by Mark—thus has the signification of resisting both forms of vulnerability, susceptibility to "internalized homophobia" as well as to being looked at "that way," by means of a confrontational exercise in visibility, overcoming Mark's own self-consciousness while forcing the viewer not to look (that way, that is to say, in horror or disgust) but to *see*, to see what one would rather not see, whose significance one would rather not acknowledge or think about.

In short, to face it. But, because the object of vision is understood to be phobic (phobic to the subject as well as to the viewer), this implies both a form of courage on the subject's part (the courage to show) and a significant extension of the video's educational project: in addition to bearing witness through showing the writing of AIDS on the bodies of Tom and Mark, it must, as I've said, and in order for that showing to be *seen*, undertake the visual education of its viewer, an education specifically directed against homophobic denial and the horrified "look" that it produces.

The thematics of showing as a mode of witnessing implies, then, in the video, a symmetrical thematics of looking, together with a crucial distinction between looking as a mode of denial, the refusal to see, and seeing as the mode of witness, on the viewer's part, that corresponds to the video's showing. Crucial here, because it forms the qualifying test of the viewer's capacity to see, is the segment of Tom's death and the unforgettable shot of his face, rigid in death, the skin taut over the bones, with its one staring, open eye (the other obtruded by KS).

As viewers, we have known in a sense to expect this shot from the very start of the video, when Mark speaks of his own horror at discovering that a dead person's eyes do not close easily, in the two-fingered gesture familiar to us all from countless movies. *Silverlake Life* has thus situated itself specifically as other than a fiction: it represents Tom's death "live," and the eyes one tries to close pop open again. That is, they do not offer us the concession of veiling their stare, so as to provide a consoling image of repose; rather, they insist that we look back at them, unflinchingly, and see what their stare is showing us. "It was very scary to look at him the first time after he died," Mark reports. "You know, look him in the face. But I did." To look Tom in the face, as Mark has done, is scary also for the viewer, but it is necessary because it is to receive from his eyes, and to accept, as Mark does, the responsibility for continuing the task Tom has begun, pursuing the act of witness that is embodied in their stare. They require a *response*, as did Peter Hujar's staring eye, as reported by David Wojnarowicz at a similar moment: "I tried to say something to him, staring into that enormous eye" (103). So says Wojnarowicz, having instinctively photographed his dead friend's "amazing feet, his head, that open eye again" in a gesture that is both memorializing and

## An Education in Seeing

witnessing. And Mark promises: "Your friends will finish your video for you, Tom."

For the viewer the response equivalent to joining Tom's friends in the act of "finishing" the video can only take the form of learning to see, in the sense both of not turning away from what the video shows and of understanding what it cannot explicitly communicate. By the time of Tom's death we have been somewhat educated in this requirement of responsiveness by the example of the friends who visit the house as he lies dying, "to say hi," as Mark puts it (using a striking personal pronoun), "before we die." They record visual impressions: "I was surprised how quickly he had gone downhill" or "he's skinnier than I've ever seen him." Sue, though, plays a complicated— and, as Mark implies, hypocritical—game of avoidance, on the alibi that Tom needs time alone "to get ready to die": her averted gaze is itself death dealing ("like a barrage of death-notices," as Mark puts it) and thus constitutes an antimodel of the seeing that would signify a kind of survival, for Tom, by accepting the responsibility to continue his project.

Perhaps Judy, herself a photographer, provides (in contradistinction to Sue) the closest model for such a seeing gaze. She has previously taken a photo of the couple that they treasure; now—as Tom lies, thin, weak, barely conscious, the new lesions on his face (the eye but also on and around his nose) very prominent—she fetches the photograph in its frame and places it on the bed beside his face. As a metaphor for the video itself, the photo thus stands for the contrasting images of Tom's dying that the viewer is faced with. A short, but correspondingly intense, moment of absolutely silent contemplation ensues, the camera on Judy's eyes as she measures the contrast. This brief but painful pause is thus one of the video's key moments of seeing, in which the very failure of words underlines the crucial significance of responsive vision. (By contrast, MediCal sends a long, vexatious, and wordy form, exemplifying with its irrelevant questions the callous blindness of indifferent bureaucracy as—even more than Sue's avoidance—the most inappropriate of all the visits to Tom's deathbed.)

By virtue of this sequence of visits the viewer watching the final episodes of Tom's life is both assimilated to the community of his friends and interpellated in such a way as to view these moments as a sort of test, or at least an invitation to strip oneself of one's defensive reactions and attempt to see. Grimly philosophical a short while before ("The real thing is, you get what you get. [. . .] That's the life you will have lived"), Tom slips into forgetfulness, vagueness, and illusion ("which is sort of a problem," as he amiably and conversationally says, "carrying on a nice conversation"), and soon he is able only to wave at the camera. On a hot day the covers are drawn back and reveal his wasted body, as Mark explains his sense of shame at having prepared food that made Tom sick, so that he is visibly weaker. Barely audible, Tom gives his "not chipper" health bulletin. And, finally, we see his staring face, as Mark laments: "Tommy's just died," and cries: "Isn't he beautiful? He's so beautiful." It is as if the ability at least to glimpse that beauty is the final test of the viewer's capacity to see, since it appears to be associated with Mark's promise to finish the video and hence with the continuation of Tom's autobiography and the form of survival the completed video represents, its "impact" intensified by the authority of death, an impact for which another name might perhaps be beauty.

"We promise to finish the tape for you": in saying this, Mark speaks, then, not only for the group of surviving friends who will complete the video in a technical sense but also for the viewers who, by their ability to see, will accept the continuance of this project as their own responsibility and qualify, not solely as Tom's survivors, but more particularly as the inheritors of his task, the bearers of witness on his behalf.

To be Tom's survivor is thus to accept responsibility for the survival of something like Tom's spirit. This survival of Tom in symbolic or transcendental form is alluded to in the video in a number of ways. The allusion is structural in the relay of autobiographical responsibility between Tom and Mark and narrative in the story of Mary Jospin's conversion and her adoption of Mark as her "son." Thematically, Tom's survival is intertwined with the representation of Mark's own survivorhood, as in the final episodes of the video we see him carrying out the duties of grief and memory. Officialdom zips Tom's body into a white plastic bag and carries it away, leaving Mark with only a how-to book about grief sent him by his therapist, which he reads for us sardonically. We witness the memorial service, and we watch Mark receive the package containing Tom's ashes, opening it clumsily, transferring them to an urn, and spilling them a bit in the process. And, finally, Peter Friedman interviews him on camera about his survivorhood: how does it feel? He is exhausted, with his own AIDS and his own falling T-cell count on his mind ("I'm just *really beat*"); his present life is "really confusing." He discusses his modified relation both with Tom's mother and with his own father, who has written him a "surreal" letter, which Mark interprets as signaling "acknowledgment" of his relation with Tom. And then he drops a bombshell. Mark has always thought, he says, that death was "the end," but now—suddenly and unexpectedly ("Zoom!")—Tom has returned and visits him regularly. Mark has felt his presence, "leaning in" to him, "a strange energy."

Mark goes on to explain that he has attempted to free Tom to "diffuse into the universe" if he wishes to ("I'll survive without you"), only to receive the response: "You idiot, I have nothing else to do now." Tom's survival, in other words, has a determinate sense, and he retains some sort of identity. He is, nevertheless, dead, Mark adds, and he knows it. "So he's not, like, stuck here." These words are important: they resonate with the video's subtitle (*The View from Here*) and, more particularly, with a brief scene in the desert, before Tom's death, when Mark stood by the roadside with arms outstretched, wiggling his fingers in response to Tom's request for "action" and explaining: "I'm a sign, and the sign reads: 'We're here.'" There is a difference, then, between being a sign, in Mark's sense—clearly a mode of testimonial and linked to the video's thematics of showing—and the form of Tom's survival, which is invisible but consists of no longer being "stuck here" without however having "diffuse[d] into the universe."

"Tom, you're all over the place," Mark had said affectionately when the ashes spilled (where *place* is referentially imprecise but contrasts with "diffuse[d] into the universe"). That's as good a metaphor as any, perhaps, for the difference the video constructs between the order of visibility that "signs" represent—the order of *showing*, with its message: "We're here," "This is our view, from here"—and the form of *readability* (diffused not into the universe but throughout a text) that, say, a video can achieve, as the mode of its author's postmortem survival and a way of witnessing in its own right. But what mediates the difference is the viewer's willingness and ability to accept the responsibility of seeing, that is, to confront something in the object of vision that no amount of mere looking will apprehend because it asks to be read.

A certain relation of difference, but also of continuity, between visual confrontation (a matter of "being a sign") and survival, as the transcendence of signhood that signs can mediate, is thus at the very heart of the video. Two images from the final scenes capture something of this relation. When Tom's body in its white plastic shroud is slid into the back of a van and is about to be driven away, to return in the form of ashes, the camera lingers—as it earlier lingered on Judy's gaze—on the image of the shapeless white lump of Tom's body in the bag, viewed through the glass. But the image also captures the reflection of the camera itself, with Mark's head at the eyepiece, making this an image of confrontation, of the face-to-faceness of showing and seeing that being a sign entails. It is "the view from here." But also, once in a while during the harrowing scenes of Tom's dying, the camera has caught in its frame the household cat, curled up comfortably on the same bed. Now, during the final interview, as Mark explains that he has been "adopted" by Tom's mother as her son, we see a (grand)motherly image of Mary, cradling the cat in her arms.

Like Guibert's butterfly (the creature that emerges transformed from a chrysalis), the cat, which is reputed to enjoy nine lives, is a figure of metempsychosis. Tom lives on, then, in modified form, as the object of Mary's affection—an object that has as its concrete existent form not Tom (he is no longer "stuck here") but Mark and the cat. Tom's survival, in other words, is readable (although it is not visible) in the cat, embraced by Mary, and in her adoption of Mark; but Tom's death, as an act of witness—his disappearance from the universe of being here and being a sign—was the condition of this form of survival. These, then (the cat, Mark standing in for Tom), are "signs" (perhaps I should call them figures) but in a sense different from the signs—they might be called marks, with an allusion both to the name of Tom's surviving lover and to Kaposi's lesions—that can simply display, or show, their meaning. They produce significations (an effect of reading) other than their conventional signified—an effect dependent, therefore, on the interpretive intervention of a viewer capable of responding to what they show by *seeing* their significance, *reading* the marks as figures, and understanding their figuration as the signs

## An Education in Seeing

of survival that they are. Such a response is the opposite of the homophobic look that fails to see.

There is an even more resplendent image of survival, however. It occurs at the very start of the video, where its full significance tends to escape a first-time viewer. Mark's early account of his horror at discovering that Tom's eyes will not close and of the "scariness" of looking him in the face is hard to get out of one's memory (even though the corresponding image comes only later). It still lingers in the mind as we see, moments later, an image of Tom (a visibly young, healthy, smiling Tom) that Tom had made as a video greeting card for Mark on a celebratory occasion. It shows his bespectacled face, framed in a cardboard cutout in the shape of a heart and bearing the words "I love you": Tom beams with pleasure and satisfaction. In the context of what we have just heard about Tom's death, the contrast is, of course, startling, but the hint of transcendence introduced by the framing of Tom's radiant face also identifies the image as generically related to— a kind of homely caricature of—say, a Romanesque or Byzantine saint "in glory." It thus signifies other than what it shows.

And Tom's large, heavy-rimmed spectacles, framing his eyes as the cardboard heart frames his face, stay with us from this image throughout the video, as one of his homely but characteristic "attributes." They're often on his nose, at first (most memorably when he leans in to the camera to confide his anger at being denied an opportunity to rest by Mark's insistence on doing errands: "I hate being a nice guy!"). Later, after his death, they become a relic, resting on the dresser beside the urn that contains his ashes. We can read these spectacles, therefore, as signifying the video's faith in a certain ability to see, an ability assisted by, but not restricted to, optical aids like eyeglasses but also cameras and monitors or even the CAT scan equipment we see at the video's outset—the instruments, that is, of showing. It is such an ability to see that the video wishes to foster in its viewers, with the hope that it will be transformative, converting the marks of death into the figuration of a certain mode of survival through education of the viewers' vision. And it is perhaps such an education of vision that the eyeglasses, as a mode of prosthesis, most clearly signify from the start, perched as they are on a nose that we will soon see marked by lesions and framing eyes that will soon stare in death but in a face that alludes, however humbly and jokingly, to postmortem transfiguration.

*Zoom.* What, I wonder, can we make, now, of the one small word—an onomatopoeia and, as Mark uses it, more like an interjection than articulated speech—by which Mark indicates the speed and suddenness of Tom's visitations from beyond death? He employs it quite casually, but we cannot ignore its implications merely for that reason. It is a word that has colloquial currency but derives from a technical lexicon. In the technology of flying, to zoom is to change altitude, upward or downward, with great speed, swooping or soaring, climbing or diving, with a sudden increase in momentum and a concomitant release, and expenditure, of energy. In film technology a zoom shot brings an object into rapid focus, with again a very sudden decrease in distance and often an effect of the camera's swooping down and in from a height. Zooming thus effects a change in degree, but it does this so markedly that it comes to resemble a change in quality: from cruising speed to the deployment of great power, or from a visual blur to sharp focus. That is what makes it available as a metaphor of qualitative passage: a zoom might bring one back across the divide of death to survive and to visit among the living, as Tom does—but it might also stand for a qualitative improvement in perception, such as a transformation of mere looking into seeing, in the way that one can go, in one swoop, from a distanced and indistinct blur to the greatest visual precision and relief. Mark's offhand near-interjection alerts us, I think, to the metaphorics of passage—of survival, on the one hand, and of learning to see, on the other—that underlies the whole project of *Silverlake Life.*

We have noted already (at the end of chap. 3) that, between the representation of an author's dying and the act of interpretation that prolongs its witness—reading the representation as signifying " 'I' is dead" or enjoying in the present instant "the wealth of the past"—the moment of the author's death intervenes, without being itself either representable or interpretable. The overcoming of that moment on which discursivity has no purchase and the consequent survival of the authorial subject under the transformed guise of textual subjectivity are represented in Guibert as a form of haunting: the power of writing as phantom imagery. In Tom Joslin's video the equivalent metaphor is one that also has spiritualist overtones, but it is less spectral than it is technological. *Zoom* puts emphasis quite squarely on the power of technologies of representation, and especially of visual representation, to convert the homophobic "look," which puts distance between the observer and the observed, into "seeing": a readerly apprehension that responds in sympathetic, involved fashion to an authority borrowed from death and in so doing becomes capable of what we can now call *seerdom*, receiving the visitation of the erstwhile authorial subject in transformed (textual) guise.

"Zoom," from the angle of the now deceased author, is thus a mechanism of survival, one that depends, however, on the engaged— rather than phobic, evasive, or dismissive—survivorhood of viewers willing to see, that is to read, what can neither be said nor directly shown, the ultimate mystery called (the) death (of the author). Two zooms are thus in play: the textual subject can only zoom in and visit a reader whose own vision is qualified to receive that visitation— qualified, that is, by virtue of an education in seeing that makes it capable, in turn, of a zoom that reduces distance and converts unseeing blur into seeing, up-close "focus." And everything in *Silverlake Life* suggests that the quality that resists homophobic distance and denial and makes the double zoom possible, bringing about a convergence of authorial survival and readerly survivorhood, is love: most centrally the love of Tom and Mark, reiterated time and again throughout the video, but also the love that circulates among their friends and forms a community into which, finally, even the homophobic parents are integrated. Not suicide but love is the antidote to homophobia.

But the readerly act of love that ensures the survival of the textual subject is thus defined negatively, as the opposite of homophobic avoidance. The visited, seeing reader is one who is denied the option of denial and whose attention is complete, and it is this marshaling of attention that is indicated by the metaphor of the zoom shot, which figures reading as a bringing of the object into focus. But focus also points to a difference, and perhaps an incompatibility, between the readerly zoom of seeing (a function of survivorhood) and the zoom of visitation that figures the survival of textual subjectivity. For a reader's vision can be said to be focused because it is necessarily positioned: like the particular perspective of showing indicated by the video's subtitle, the readerly perspective on a text is always itself something of a view from here, not in the relativizing sense of one text "viewed" from different angles but because reading as a construction of "the" text is always specifically mediated by unexamined assumptions. Thus, it frames, selects, and orders the materials on which it imposes a particular coherence that another reading, differently mediated, would not reproduce.

Tom, though, as we learn from Mark, is—after his death—no longer "stuck here": without being "diffuse[d] into the universe," he is no longer the subject of a positioned view. That is the difference between Tom as (former) subject of an *énoncé* he was able to control and "Tom" as the name might be pressed into service to designate the form of textual subjectivity into which he has died, that is, the subjectivity of *énonciation*. But such (unpositioned) textual subjectivity, definitionally, cannot be exhausted by any single, inevitably positioned and so "focused," act of interpretation. Our readings, in that sense, are always misreadings, however well intentioned, attentive, and even engaged they may be: they are not necessarily wrong, but they are inescapably constrained and constraining, in a way that admits of the possibility of other constrained and constraining positions and other readings. Thus, it is indeed the very fact of their "attentiveness"—to the extent that attentiveness implies focus and so position—that militates against their ability to realize the apparently limitless potential for signification that textual subjectivity has gained from the death of its authorial subject (i.e., the loss of a controlling position, or view from here, embodied in the intentionality of an *énoncé*).

In other words, the survivorhood of the reader, without which there can be no textual survival of the dying author, simultaneously ensures the inadequacy and unsatisfactoriness of that survival, not only in the sense that the reader's position necessarily differs from the original positionality of the authorial subject, the one writing as "a living dead," the other reading as a survivor, but also because *no* positioned readerly perspective can realize the full significance of "unpositioned" textuality or respond adequately to a subjectivity that is no longer stuck here and tied to a view. Reading, therefore, is subject in this analysis to a double bind, one that makes it simultaneously an expression of love and an anxious practice: the reader can neither not read (avoidance is forbidden the reader, who is required to focus) nor yet respond adequately and appropriately to the demand, for an *unlimited* reading, that is made by the textual visitation.

The clutter and messiness of the Silverlake house—the household objects, the furniture, the equipment that lie about in disorderly profusion and often fill the frame of the image—is thus not

## An Education in Seeing

only an indicator of the "live"-ness of the representation (chap. 2). It also represents a challenge to the focus without which there is no readerly seeing, a reminder of the impossibility of responding adequately to a text that—borrowing its authority from death (not being subject to authorial control of its meaning)—is theoretically a site of communicational "noise" and admits therefore of a limitless multiplicity of potential, and not necessarily convergent, readings. Such untidiness situates reading as a constraining, tidying operation. But equally, and conversely, the fullness of the house, with its human and animal residents and the friends and family who stop by or visit—another form of clutter—signals not only, in general terms, the power of community against disease and death, including death-dealing homophobia, but also the act of love the video's viewers are invited to accomplish, in learning to see what it is showing and joining its community: that is, in becoming its readers and ensuring the survival of its textual subject.

That there is an incompatibility between the invitation that is issued and the conditions of success that are imposed on it—the invitation to read and the possibility of an adequate reading—does not prevent the demand from being formulated, then, or its challenge from being accepted. It means only that the conditions of witnessing, as a discourse that borrows its authority from death, are inevitably anxiogenic and that they are anxiogenic on both sides of the authorial-readerly divide. Will the representation of my dying, can it, find a readership capable of ensuring its survival? asks the author. Does my survivorhood necessarily disqualify me as an adequate respondent to a text that bears witness, in its unlimited readability, to the fact of death? asks the reader.

AIDS, then, it seems, will have been—among many other things and inasmuch as it poses the problem of bearing witness—an epidemic of rhetorical anxiety: anxiety about being read, anxiety about reading. The thematics of visitation in both Guibert and Joslin points clearly enough to that double anxiety: how to die into a text that will visit my survivors; how, as a survivor, to respond adequately to textual visitation. One of the merits of Eric Michaels's *Unbecoming*, though, is to have explicitly, without recourse to the metaphor of visitation (with its inevitably supernatural connotations), framed the problem of AIDS witnessing as a problem in rhetoric and to have defined that problem as a problem in survival through the transmission not of a message or even of a surviving textual subjectivity but of rhetorical anxiety itself.

How to ensure a mode of textual survival such that authorial anxiety about being read will live on in the form of readers' anxiety about the adequacy of their readerly response? That is the question that animates Michaels's writing. And, accordingly, Michaels's figure of survival, his metaphorics of passage, will not be spectral imagery or zooming visitations but—exactly as his rhetorical preoccupations would suggest—a tongue. A tongue marked by KS lesions, as both the writing of AIDS and the sign of death. But a tongue extended.

# 5

## Anxious Reading: Eric Michaels's *Unbecoming*

Ill people whose unaccommodating behavior earns them the reputation of being "difficult patients" are a trial to their caregivers and friends. There is a sense, though, in which the practices of AIDS witnessing, to the extent that they represent a refusal to give up and go quietly from the scene (as so many would like AIDS "victims" to do), function as a social correlative of the refractory performance turned in by so-called difficult patients. In its very title Eric Michaels's AIDS diary signals its project of making "the writing of AIDS" a site in which "unbecoming," as the disintegration of an individual body and the disappearance of a person—the death of an author—can become an occasion for the production of social discomfort through an equally unbecoming rhetorical performance. The purpose and effect of Michaels's writing is to deprive readers who, as survivors, may be prone to believe themselves unaffected by the epidemic of any possibility of equanimity or complacency, by putting them under something like the stress suffered by the friends of a difficult patient. The text thus offers an opportunity to reflect on AIDS witnessing as it is modeled by the difficult patient performance and to examine the rhetorical stakes of such an exercise in unbecoming(ness).

Peter Hujar, in *Close to the Knives,* is described by David Wojnarowicz as a difficult patient (see "Living Close to the Knives" 84–110). Wojnarowicz tells, for example, how he and a friend, Anita, drove Peter to Long Island to consult a quack doctor offering a miracle cure for AIDS. Peter is too weak to take the train, as he threatens to do, and so is completely dependent on his friends' help, yet he behaves abominably, complaining that there must be a faster way to get there when there isn't, insisting on stopping on the freeway to pee, refusing to be touched although he can't get out of the car without assistance. "'Don't touch me.' 'Peter, I have to touch you to help you out.' 'Don't touch me it hurts'" (91). The painful journey winds up with a meal in a diner:

> He barely touched his food, staring out the window and saying, "America is such a beautiful country—don't you think so?" I was completely exhausted from the day, emotionally and physically, and looking out the window at the enormous collage of high-tension wires, blinking stoplights, shredded used-car banners, industrial tanks and masses of humanity zipping about in automobiles just depressed me. The food we had in front of us looked like it had been fried in an electric chair. And watching my best friend dying while eating a dead hamburger left me speechless. I couldn't answer. Anita couldn't either. He got angry again. "Neither of you would know what I'm talking about . . ." Finally I said, "Peter, we're very tired. Let's go home." (98)

At home Peter withdraws to his bed and angrily dismisses his friends. "Later, talking on the telephone with Vince, I heard that Peter had talked with him minutes after Anita and I had left his house and Peter said, 'I don't understand it, they just put me in bed and rushed out'" (99). For the patient exasperation arises from a kind of *nec tecum nec sine te* (neither with nor without you) relation to his friends, who are both indispensable and a constant reminder of his loss of independence and agency; for the friends anxiety arises from being put in a perpetual double bind, their help being required but simultaneously dismissed as inappropriate. I want to redescribe that dynamic, in what follows, as the rhetorical interaction that generates the situation I call "anxious reading."

The point of *Unbecoming*, in the first instance, is to give an account of why Eric Michaels, in life, felt constrained to adopt the persona of the difficult patient as well as to transcribe that role into the writing of his dying. Trained as an anthropologist and having worked for five years among people (the Warlpiri) who, like many Australian Aboriginal groups, name individuals according to their classificatory social position and understand identity in terms of responsibility for the preservation of specific cultural information (stories, songs, designs, rituals, including the maintenance of sacred sites), he was professionally predisposed to understand individual biography as socially significant. To be gay, therefore, as gayness has been lived in Western countries since Stonewall, is, for Michaels, to occupy a social position of oppositionality, and to be infected with AIDS in 1987 is to be under attack from the social forces—not solely homophobia but a range of pressures toward conformity, orderliness, and homogeneity—to which open and "liberated" gayness is an affront. AIDS is, so to speak, in alliance with those forces, and it is the PWA's duty, therefore, to fight back for as long as he lives and, if possible, to ensure—since it is social issues, not individual destinies, that are at stake—that resistance is carried on beyond the death of the individual sufferer. In that way, although AIDS destroys individuals, the more important factor of social resistance will be preserved. The function of the diary, therefore, will be to provide evidence of Michaels's personal refusal to accept victimhood and to go quietly but also to ensure the continuance of the spirit of recalcitrance his battle represents in the future society of which Michaels, as a person, will no longer be a member.

But out of such reasoning comes, for Michaels as a writer, a kind of *nec tecum nec sine te* relation toward the social persona he attributes to himself and the social agency he wishes the diary to enjoy: without it he dies absolutely, and the spirit of resistance disappears, but with it his personality and individual agency count for nothing. The difficult patient role he adopts could plausibly be read as an attempt to resolve this tension: a classificatory identity in the disciplinary society of the hospital (and beyond) but one that individualizes the patient as one who has too strong a personality to blend into the crowd. But the tension surfaces also in the form of what Michaels calls paranoia. For what exactly justifies an individual in the view that significant social forces are doing battle in his person? The general view seems to be to the opposite effect, and such "paranoia" therefore functions as an uncomfortable confirmation of the patient's individual status, holding views that make him the only one out of step. The diary as difficult patient performance—inevitably an irrational rhetorical position to occupy—thus comes to coexist with the diary as a site of informal, but rational, social analysis, designed to prove the proposition that individual positions are socially constituted and that the difficult patient's irrational oppositionality is not just a sign of individual craziness, therefore, because it is socially justified. Michaels, in this way, is keeping paranoia at bay. For the reader, however, all this translates into the paradox that, in a book that lays claim to purely social agency, a voice speaks that is recognizably and inimitably personal: the supposedly "social," rhetorical subject is that of an unusually vivid (and likable) performance of "personality," the performance of a difficult patient who is not altogether comfortable in his role.

But on the side of reading an anxiety is thus generated, or can be generated, that corresponds symmetrically to paranoia and the struggle against paranoia, on the side of writing. For, in responding in this way to the voice of Michaels's personality is it not possible, and indeed probable, that I am simultaneously betraying the social agency the text is anxious to exercise and of which, now that the author is dead, I as its reader have become the bearer? But equally, in realizing the text as a social agent only (supposing I could do that), would I not be displaying culpable indifference to the death of the individual author, on whose disappearance the purely social identity of the text depends? To realize the text as an agent of social oppositionality, independent of the individual personality of the author that speaks in it, would be an act of complacency equivalent to the social delinquency of failure to mourn the dead.

This particular difficulty, of being able to read legitimately neither for purely social significance nor for personality, corresponds, I want to suggest, to a more general definition of the double bind that is normally and definitionally placed on readers, who are required, by the death of the author in its theoretical sense, to realize textual significances that transcend authorial intention and control but can do so only under limits of positionality that make reading comparable to an interpersonal communication. But it also suggests that the anxiety of reading is a function, in the long run, of the essential paradox of culture, which is that human beings are its agents in a double sense: without our agency, as persons, there is no transmission or production of culture, yet culture works through us, as its agents, in ways we can neither fathom nor control, to produce a history that makes a mockery of all individual claims to the privilege of agency. Michaels's text, with its authorial paranoia, on one side, and the readerly anxiety it produces, on the other, might be viewed in this light as a singularly self-conscious enactment, in the mode of worry, of this paradox of culture and the problematic it generates of the relation of individuals to history.

*Anxious Reading*

But for now, and in this context, it is the symmetry of the rhetorical relation of authorial paranoia and readerly anxiety that I want to stress: to the *nec tecum sine te* of writing corresponds the "damned if you do, damned if you don't" of reading. This symmetry signals a difference between the imaginary of representation and communication that is at work in *La pudeur ou l'impudeur* and *Silverlake Life*— which include a transcendental dimension in their figuring of communication across death and writerly survival through reading—and Michaels's vision of the ability of essential social relations to survive the death of persons and hence of writing and reading as purely discursive phenomena. Such phenomena are without transcendence, but, governed by a rhetoric that reproduces something of the agonistics—of ordering and resistance to order—that defines Michael's view of social relations in general, they are traversed also by an anxiety about the relation of the personal to the social that derives from the cultural paradox. His figure for the passage that marks the difference, bounded by the author's death, between writing and reading is therefore not a figure of other-worldly visitation, involving spectral imagery or zooming, but, as I've said and as it will be necessary to explore at much greater length, an extended tongue—the protruding tongue, marked by the writing of AIDS in the form of cancerous lesions, in the photograph of the dying author that serves as a frontispiece to the volume.

Such an image is a figure of connection, representing the power of discourse to survive the death of its authorial subject in order to remain rhetorically active in the world of those who survive. But it is also a figure of impudence, recalcitrance, and resistance, representing the power of that discourse to survive as an act of social provocation capable of unsettling the survivors, its readers. The greatest danger, for a resisting text, is that it survive its author's demise only to be read complacently, in a way that fails to realize its resistant potential and so confirms the victory of the ordering forces that are responsible, in the form of AIDS, for the death of the author. The necessary unsettling of the reader is figured, therefore, by the provocatively outstretched tongue. But reading—this is an axiom I've already alluded to and to which I will return—cannot fail to fall short of the textual demands that are made of it and so can't fail to confirm the author's death and hence the power of social order to contain resistance—and that is, I suggest, another reason for the dying author's last gesture to be a defiant one, but an act now of personal defiance, in the face of the inevitable loss of individual agency that will result from his death.

In the end, then, it is the reality of an individual's death that must be faced, given the strictly immanent character of Michaels's view of things: it is that reality that haunts both authorial paranoia and readerly anxiety and makes the scenario of survival to which *Unbecoming* (nevertheless) subscribes a singularly dubious one. Ultimately, the symmetry between the side of writing and the side of reading in communication, the mirror image each form of worry presents to the other, derives from the fact that the death of the author, which defines the entry of a text into the moment of reading, is also and already—indeed always already—palpable in the moment of writing, understood as the site where the rights of the personal surrender to those of the social, in the form of textuality. And AIDS can thus become the sign both of that unbecoming into writing, figured by the disintegration of the individual body, and of the reality of death as it (pre-) occurs in life. Not so much a disease in itself as the precondition for the attack of opportunistic diseases of variable severity, ranging from the "merely" incommoding and humiliating to the life threatening, it is, as Michaels puts it, "the disease of a thousand rehearsals" (139/94), and the rehearsals are rehearsals for death. And because, for Michaels, it is one manifestation of a general feature of social existence that he finds oppressive, it joins forces with a host of other contingencies, ranging from the "merely" irritating to the debilitating, to signify the preposthumous presence of death in the AIDS sufferer's life: "It's the specificities that wipe us out in the end" (156/106). It becomes easy, therefore, at certain moments, for the sufferer to imagine he is already dead: "I'm starting to have this odd sense of being at my own funeral. [. . .] I lie in bed feeling like I'm peering out of my own coffin" (146/99). So that his life prior to death comes to mirror, symmetrically, an experience of postmortem survival.

Under such dire circumstances two reactions are possible. One is the thought of suicide, the simple desire to give up and abandon the struggle to resist. The other is the opposite: to take advantage of the similarity of the preposthumous condition of living with AIDS as a dying subject of writing and the posthumous condition of having died into readability from AIDS, in order to bring about a certain continuity of survival, between the author resisting death and the text that will go on, after his death, to resist the social forces for which AIDS stands. This, in Michaels's telling metaphor, becomes a matter of "stage-managing" one's death, with a clear implication of rhetorical performance and indeed of calculation for a particular effect. For dying of AIDS and the writing of one's dying require management so as to produce the effect of "resistance," to the extent that they function as a denial of the urge to give up and to submit to death, which would be a kind of suicide. And one stage-manages one's dying, then—and the writing of one's dying—so as to stage-manage one's posthumous existence, as the difficult patient who dies living on, by virtue of a fractious journal, in the form of a socially effective text of resistance.

The difference between the two phases seems minimal, just the little matter of the author's actual death, which is already such a palpable reality in his preposthumous existence. Thus, on May 28, 1988, in a moment of severe discouragement, Eric Michaels wrote:

> I'm sure death itself is the simplest thing in the world. The choice seems merely to be this: to arrange everything, to maintain a morbid fantasy of control, or to simply give up and let go. The latter looks to me more and more appealing. (138/93)

But the existence of the diary, of course, with its final entry dated August 10, 1988, just two weeks before the author's death supervened on August 24, is testimony to the strength of his commitment to "the morbid fantasy of control." And my reading of it, already some years after his death, is evidence that, whatever "control" might actually signify in this circumstance (which is the question my essay turns on), Michaels's fantasy was not a pure illusion.

That fantasy, of controlling a certain posthumous survival, subtends all the thinking about genre in *Unbecoming* and all the speculation about publishing, finding, and reaching a readership—the definitional question of conceiving an AIDS diary (written for whom? and from what position? following which models? in relation to which adjacent genres?) and the closely related pragmatic question of turning a supposedly intimate and personal genre (the private diary) into an agency of witness, capable of exerting significant social effect. Taken together, these concerns do not only form a new area of worry in the text, one that links authorial paranoia to readerly anxiety by speculating about how to effect that link. Michaels's thinking and questioning also amount to the most extended reflection I know of on what is at stake in the writing of AIDS, understood as the "stage management" of an author's death in the interests of a politics of resistance, that is, as a double act (pre- and postmortem) of witness that is an "act" in a double sense: an action whose effect is dependent on facticity.

The undeviating principle running through these reflections is the desire to convert, through the stage management that is representation, a form of defeat—the unbecoming of an author afflicted with AIDS and beset by social hostility—into the possibility not, of course, of victory or triumph but of continued resistance (that possibility being itself a kind of victory). Under what conditions of stage management, through what writerly agency, can a tale of disintegration become an unbecoming social gesture, the rhetorical equivalent of poking out one's tongue in the reader's face? When, in the opening sentences of his first entry (Sept. 9, 1987), Eric Michaels describes his recently appeared lesions as "morphemes" and imagines stringing them together into sentences that would form a story—"a narrative trajectory, a plot outline" (23/3)—we can suppose, then, that the story he has in mind is the story framed by that question: the conversion of his personal unbecoming into something more durably and productively, because rhetorically, unbecoming.

Let us begin by noting the presence in *Unbecoming* of an intermittent poetics of lamentation, which can be read as a kind of stylistic harking back to very ancient historical strata: those of a certain Jewish tradition, biblical and diasporic, of survival—and of survival under the direst of circumstances. But it also has overtones of queenly "bitching" and perhaps even of what, in Australia, is known as "whingeing."

> I've been ragged and paranoid all week. Fevers and sweats coming and going and some odd lung thing that's scary. My tumours itch and seem to be developing psoriatic complications or something. It's been raining as long as I can recall; everything is mould, mould, mould. The kitchen is filled with flying weevils. The toilet is backed up. My neighbour has taken up the saxophone and tries to play hits from *The*

*Sound of Music* all day. I can't sleep and can't do anything but. I wake up repeatedly in the middle of the night with the horrors. I don't even want to call anybody. I have no interest in working and I haven't even been pursuing my immigration business responsibly. My physician seems to have deserted me. My conviction that the world I perceive corresponds to anybody else's is slipping. Maybe I died in November and this is some awful postmortem fantasy I inhabit now? (118–19/80)

I don't quote this passage as characteristic (the book is very varied in subject matter and style, containing passages of social analysis, autobiographical reflection, and academic polemic as well as, or as part of, its reporting from the AIDS front). I quote it as indicative. The world Eric Michaels inhabits is purely immanent (no butterflies or cats à la Guibert or Joslin); it is hostile and debilitating; and the appropriate response elicited by distressing contingencies does not entail displays of heroism in the stoic mode or rhetorical discretion and a sense of *pudeur*. Instead of serene courage or restraint, what gets displayed with some ostentation, through rhetorical devices of accumulation and excess, is worry and paranoia, even a certain self-pity (mitigated by humor), and a spirit of complaint. A whole heap of particularities, from scary symptoms to weevils in the kitchen and an irritating neighbor, weigh on the protesting spirit and motivate perfectly unjust accusations (the physician's alleged defection), depression and apathy (failure to look after important business), a sense of isolation and incipient madness (the discrepancy between subjective vision and that of others), and morbid fantasy ("Maybe I died in November . . ."), and these in turn furnish further subjects of complaint.

The refusal one can see here of any mitigating or idealizing vision, although it is itself anything but serene, is in line with Michaels's dismissal, in another place, of the *sentimental* in the name of what he calls first principles: "At least one reason for publishing this journal is to counter the sentimentalised narrative that seems to be all that San Francisco has been able to produce about this sequence; and to reconfirm first principles" (144/97). I don't know what the target of the San Francisco jibe is, but the passage requires us, therefore, to attempt to elucidate the first principles that lie behind its unwillingness to sentimentalize the experience of AIDS and why the AIDS crisis requires them to be reconfirmed. I'll stress the way these principles can be thought to be performed in the passage's rhetoric, understood as a mode of resistance that is embodied in the persona of its speaker, "ragged and paranoid" as he may be. Indeed, it is the relation between lamentation and paranoia, and the sense in which both relate to resistance, that I particularly want to try to understand.

Michaels's first principles, as I've already in fact suggested, are three in number, and each requires an unsentimental approach: there is a principle of immanence, a principle of resistance, and a principle of continuity or survival. Not only is the world a hostile place and AIDS a dire affliction, but there is no beyond. Any "postmortem" life will therefore be figurative—"some awful [. . .] fantasy I inhabit now," the sense that AIDS produces, as "the disease of a thousand rehearsals" (139/94), of having outlived oneself and of experiencing death while still alive. Or, if it is genuinely posthumous (the author's death being not fantasy but reality), it can only entail survival in a strictly immanent sense, that is, in the form of mourning as a matter of social practices and arrangements for dealing with the death of a member of society, including the disposition of property and (of particular interest to Michaels) of intellectual property: the survival in collective memory of a textual and social "self."

The second and third principles therefore entail the necessity, short of giving up, going under, and abandoning meaningful forms of survival, to "stage-manage [one's] own posthumosity" (152/103), ensuring by this means that there will be some survival of the will to resist, some continuity between the grievously assailed subject of pre-posthumous postmortem experience and the social participant a text can be as a posthumous survivor of its author's actual death—in other words, between a certain performance of unbecoming and an unbecoming social performance. I submit that the rhetoric of the passage I just quoted—its inspired kvetching, its performance of exasperation—is part and parcel of the stage management of that double (present and future) "posthumosity."

In this project, as I've also already proposed, the ability to stage-manage (a recurring metaphor in *Unbecoming*) is clearly crucial: a certain factitious rhetorical performance is the *only* alternative (short of suicide) to the depredations of AIDS and the forces it is aligned with, that is, to the threat of being reduced to such a degree of passivity that there will be no spirit of resistance to survive posthumously. That is why it is important, in the lamenting passage, which in its *énoncé* seems to record a sense of defeat, for us as its readers to catch (in the *énonciation*) the tone—a bit campy, humorous, and wry—that indicates a surviving resistant subjectivity and produces Michaels, as subject of his writing, as anything but a defeated figure, despite the Jobian list of ills that beset Michaels the PWA. But because *paranoia* names in the text the sense of isolation, as well as the excessive rhetoric, that also characterizes such a resisting subject ("My conviction that the world I perceive corresponds to anyone else's is slipping"), it is helpful also, in understanding the passage's embattled tone, to have some understanding of the circumstances that nourished the historical Eric Michaels's "paranoid" vision of a situation that anyone would have to agree was objectively dire.

A United States citizen, he was dying in semi-isolation in Brisbane (Australia), a city that came to represent for him the worst of everything that he was facing. As an active participant in the New York gay liberation movement in 1969–72, he was now "without direct involvement in the gay world" (79/43); for five years (1982–87) he had been closely involved, as an anthropologist, in the life of the Warlpiri community at Yuendumu (Central Australia). There was thus a double contrast with his Brisbane life, in which he felt "comparatively alone" and "minimally connected" (55/26). On the evidence of the diary itself he had the support of numerous relatively distant friends but could rely on little on-the-spot help. He seems furthermore to have been virtually estranged from his "crazy" family in the United States and concludes bleakly, at one point, that "if my family is to take any major responsibility for my care, we will have to invent that family" (74/39). It would not be surprising, under such conditions, if the daily aggravations of a life in which nothing ever seemed to go right—a common perception, I know—but also some less common difficulties, such as the bureaucratic harassment of an Immigration Department intent on deporting him and the disciplinary regime or "Foucauldian horror show" (25/4) of the hospital, began to loom very large and very discouragingly: whence the bitter conclusion finally expressed toward the end that "it's the specificities that wipe us out in the end" (156/106). Paranoia, or more accurately the suspicion of being paranoid, would have reinforced that discouragement by adding a sense of mental isolation to the social and geographical isolation of the sufferer.

But, as we've seen (it is a matter of first principle), *giving up* is itself tantamount to being *wiped out*, an acceptance of the likelihood of disappearing without trace, and one must therefore not give up, even if one's resistance is reduced to lamentation, that is, to complaining about one's impotence and inability to resist. And in that context paranoia can become an unexpected ally, because in an odd way paranoia itself, together with the ability to worry about being paranoid, confirms not only one's isolation but also one's status as a resisting subject. One needs to resist because one feels threatened, but the very fact of feeling threatened—whether it is a paranoid belief or not—guarantees one's difference with respect to the unsuspicious norm of social beings, and thus grounds one's fear and need to resist. Furthermore, paranoid anxiety and anxiety about one's possible paranoia are themselves, in the end, indistinguishable. As Michaels points out (61/30), the very question: "am I paranoid?" which sounds like a manifestation of rationality, is already a paranoid question, while, as Freud was aware, there is no reliable way to distinguish paranoia, as *delirium interpretandi*, from legitimately suspicious (social or) psychoanalytic theorizing. In the end, then, it is the anxiety itself that qualifies the resister, so that resisting threat, worrying about being paranoid, asserting the situation of danger one believes oneself to be in, and producing reasoned justifications for such assertions all turn out to be part of a single continuum of suspicious(ly) self-defensive behavior, which might in the end be no more than a sign of simple good sense. Paranoia asks undecidably: is it just me, or do they really want to kill me? It asserts the indissolubility of private terrors and social realities.

So, in *Unbecoming* one encounters assertions that certainly sound paranoid enough: Michaels describes his position as a PWA as "a way of dying which I, but maybe only I, believe has elements of murder" (53/25), and adds later, without the carefully restrictive clause but with a parallel acknowledgment of possible illusion: "I feel they can smell me now, like an injured member of the pack.... And they go for me, the sons of bitches, they go for the throat" (60/30). "I'm again impressed," he writes again of the same hospital—clearly his model for the whole social world—"with how the place [...] tries to enforce passivity (unto death, I dare say) so that to get any work done I have to work around and against the realisation that I'm in a place that wants to kill me (even as my doctors—some of them—try to save me)" (147/99). But one also reads an elaborate social analysis that underpins and accounts for Michaels's vision of the world in general, and the hospital in particular, as hostile, drawing out the sense in which the disciplinary world of "Foucauldian horror show" can be understood as life threatening: a site of preposthumous experience that needs now to be represented not just as a living death (which suggests passivity) but as an extended murder—the experience of being actively, if slowly, killed and of having therefore, not only to resist but to keep up one's resistance over a long period of time. And consequently, when Michaels writes to a friend, in almost coldly theoretical terms, that "the hardest part [of being in hospital] really is maintaining resistance to the institutional discourses of the public hospital system so as to retain some dignity, assurance and self-definition" (141/95), the sentence can be taken equally to support statements of the type "I'm in a place that wants to kill me" and lengthy passages of plausible social analysis that draw connections between Foucauldian disciplinarity and modes of ultimately lethal oppression.

Paranoid anxiety and anxiety about paranoia, including defensive demonstrations that paranoia is not involved, thus join forces as essential constituents of a discourse of resistance. In the passage of lamentation I began with, both anxieties are present, one in the long list of distressing contingencies, the other in the anxious observation "My conviction that the world I perceive corresponds to anyone else's is slipping." And they are coterminous in the opening sentence, "I've been ragged and paranoid all week," which (in its *énoncé*) acknowledges the anxiety of paranoia as real, while the fact of its enunciation implies self-diagnosis from a supposedly nonparanoid, or rational, position. Lamentation is thus motivated by paranoid perceptions of the world as unconditionally hostile but includes paranoia as one of the things it is necessary to lament and hence as part of the hostility lamentation attempts to resist. And resistance to AIDS has a similar and similarly anxious structure: it is motivated, in paranoid fashion, by the excessive significance it accords a disease understood to embody a fearsome social phenomenon—the fact of oppression— while it takes the form of a social diagnosis intended to dispel the judgment "I am paranoid" but only by justifying theoretically the fear and sense of threat originally thought paranoid.

I think the difficult patient's performance that Michaels adopts in and out of hospital, and embodies also in his diary as a rhetorical performance, can be best understood as a product of the kind of anxiety, the anxiety of resistance, conveyed by the lamenting passage and as a way of giving each component—social, individual, paranoid, nonparanoid—of resisting discourse its due. To be a difficult patient is an alternative to paranoia, since it corresponds to a known and acknowledged, and so legitimate, category in the orderly and ordering world of the hospital, itself metaphoric of the AIDS patient's world in general. But it registers a distinctly paranoid response to that world, viewed as a place where it is natural to assume that, rather than healing me, they want to kill me. And the difficult patient embodies, like paranoia itself, the problematics of resistance to the social when the resister is socially constituted and thus occupies a social "slot": on the one hand, why resist? but, on the other, how to do anything else than resist? Measured against the weight of the social, resistance is a role to be played and a rather desperate one—the role of the "individual" and a matter of "stage-management." Yet it is itself nothing other than a social role, the role of resister, which means that it is experienced simultaneously as the deepest urge of one's personality. Why, similarly, should a gay PWA resist AIDS, when it is so easy to go under? Because resisting is what gayness, as a social phenomenon, is all about. In that sense the gay PWA has no option but to be a difficult patient.

Michaels's anxiety of resistance has generic implications that it is also necessary for us to consider, since it is genre that organizes the interactions of text and reader. In general terms AIDS diaries, while their "storylessness" is well adapted to the temporal experience characteristic of AIDS as a syndrome (its day-by-dayness, intermittency, and unpredictability), are less obviously welcoming to the narrative of resistance and survival that underlies the project of AIDS witness, and the adaptation of the diary as a private journal of self-examination to the purposes of witnessing has thus led to a range of generic solutions. In some cases (Barbedette) the diary is published as a *Nachlass*, fragments found among the author's papers; more self-consciously, Pascal de Duve frames his account of the sublimity of being "writ-

Anxious Reading

ten" by HIV as a *journal de bord* or seagoing log, activating the poetics of voyaging. Video makers, to judge by the examples of Guibert and Joslin, turn spontaneously to the "home movies" model (as opposed, e.g., to the documentary). Pioneers of the genre, writing like Michaels relatively early in the epidemic and with some sense of cultural isolation, are perhaps particularly exercised by such questions: Alain Emmanuel Dreuilhe, writing in New York a text in French that was published in Paris in 1987, makes obsessive reference to war movies and military history for the model of combativity toward the virus his diary seeks to respect and enact. And Eric Michaels, who found the diarists available to him as models (Joe Orton, Anne Frank, Anaïs Nin) unhelpful, turns—perhaps for reassurance?—to familiar generic models: the legal model of the will and the, to him, habitual academic model of the position paper. The will responds to anxiety about the survival of his text, given in particular that, "as far as I can tell, I have only intellectual property to dispense" (32/10), while the principle of (paranoid) resistance implies that his document—diary and will—will also be a sort of manifesto, or *prise de position*.

These two generic responses, furthermore, are allied in that each constitutes the defense of a "position" that is experienced as *threatened*. The position paper responds to and simultaneously enacts the anxiety associated with paranoia, the fear that they want to kill me associated with the fear that the fear that they want to kill me is a paranoid fear. The will responds to the threat to survival, and specifically intellectual survival, that is represented for Michaels, as the position paper explains, not only by AIDS as a terminal disease but also by the set of oppressive social forces that AIDS is aligned with. It is against these forces that the will asserts an authority borrowed, in Benjamin's phrase, from death and hence stronger than any lethal force: the legal "last will and testament" is indeed the prime case of such discursive authority. But it does so here under particular circumstances that, in Michaels's (possibly paranoid?) perception, singularly jeopardize the recourse to such legal authority and require his will not only to guarantee the survival of his intellectual property but also to consist itself of an intellectual demonstration: "My will, it seems, will be a position paper" (32/10). In the end the will and the position paper are inseparably linked, then, indeed indistinguishable, because for the diary to have the character and function of a will (enjoying postmortem authority) it needs to combat threatening social forces through an analysis that both justifies resistance to them and constitutes an example of such resistance. But, to such general insecurity about the present and future status of his writing, Michaels's status among the Warlpiri of Yuendumu added a particular twist that can be seen to overdetermine his recourse to the diary as will and the will as position paper.

As a principled anthropologist, he had accorded the Warlpiri people among whom he worked rights of veto over the publication of his writing so that they could oversee its accuracy and appropriateness. But the Warlpiri, among whom Michaels had earned an identity (including a classificatory name) as a member of the community, are like most Aboriginal groups in their social response to death. They "maintain elaborate, protracted mourning ceremonies. As dramatic as these are, they involve a contradiction in that, upon death, an individual's property, image, even name, must be obliterated. [. . .] Songs and designs belonging to the deceased exit the repertoire, sometimes for generations" (31/9). Suppose, then, Michaels worries, that the Warlpiri insist, after his death, on the obliteration of his diary and with it all hope of survival for his project of social resistance? An ugly argument over the illustration of an article on Warlpiri art, in the journal *Art & Text*, which members of the community wish to censor because it includes phallic graffiti, supervenes later (101–3/59–61, 105/62, 109/64) to suggest that a Warlpiri ban on *Unbecoming* is not an implausible eventuality. The problem poses an interesting cultural question, one of those radical contradictions between Western and Aboriginal law that are (especially for the Aboriginal minority) a frequently lived reality in Australia. But the point of affirming *Unbecoming*'s status as a kind of will, then—a document for which Warlpiri culture obviously has no place and so automatically subject to Western jurisdiction—is clearly to ensure, in the first instance, the material survival of this piece of "intellectual property," as a first but indispensable step in its eventually reaching, and affecting, a readership. "I am not, nor have I ever imagined myself to be, a Warlpiri Aboriginal," Michaels carefully records (32/10), with an eye to future legal determinations (and an implicit allusion to the McCarthy hearings).

But, of course, an anxiety remains, since there is genuine ambiguity, if only because a will *is* meaningless in Warlpiri terms. And the ambiguity is reinforced because the Warlpiri involvement in the *Art*

*& Text* incident shows some of them to be sensitive to what Michaels calls a Tidy Town mentality. This derives in his account, via Christianity, from the white Australian mentality of tidiness—figured by Brisbane and exemplified by the hospital—that Michaels believes is destroying him and about which more will be said soon. For, will or no will, there is thus some real danger of an alliance of interests against the publication of *Unbecoming* after his death, which is why it becomes essential for the diary, in addition to its function as a will but also so as to ensure that it enjoys that function, to incorporate a position paper. It is indispensable for it to identify in advance and to critique, and hence to attempt to forestall, the dangers of the tidying mentality that, whether on the Warlpiri side or the white Australian side, or on both, threatens the diary's survival and "posthumosity."

It is fair to assume that homosexuality, and hence homophobia, lie at the heart of this whole issue. Michaels could scarcely have been "out" to the Warlpiri without prejudicing his work with, for, and among them: his death from AIDS and the diary's frankness about his sexuality could not fail to come as a shock in Yuendumu. At the same time, gayness as a social manifestation is, in his analysis, an emancipatory movement that, since the time of Stonewall, has been counteracted and virtually destroyed by repressive tendencies that are identified in his thinking with tidiness, on the one hand, and AIDS, on the other (AIDS is an agency of orderliness tidying disorderly social manifestations like gayness out of existence). Michaels understands his gayness, therefore, as a social persona that was culturally defined, in this context, by the appearance in 1969 on the social scene of a "public rather than a private form" of homosexuality (28/7), that is, of liberationist gayness as opposed to closeted homosexuality, understood as a regrettable deviance. (He appears not to have taken into account the sense in which the closet is itself a social institution.) By the same reasoning, the Eric Michaels who in 1987 has begun to display the symptoms of AIDS ("I watched these spots on my legs announce themselves over a period of weeks" [23/3]) is similarly a social entity ("this is why I have AIDS, because it is now on the cover of *Life*, circa 1987" [29/7]).

Or, more accurately, he has become a divided social entity, a site of struggle between opposed forces, his resistance to the disease and all it signifies—those general forces of repression with which it is in alliance—being itself not a purely personal affair but a social resistance, something like the necessary survival into the late 1980s of the heady oppositionality of 1969–72. At stake in the posthumous survival of *Unbecoming* (as well as in Michaels's maintenance of a resistant spirit up to his death) is therefore the social survival—the future availability to reading—of writing that will continue to represent the principle of oppositionality, signified by gayness, that in 1987 appears to be in a process of unbecoming, of disintegration under the brutal and dangerous attack of the forces of tidiness. That's why it is not enough for the diary to be testimonial, as a kind of will; the will must itself constitute a counterattack on tidiness, having the function of a position paper.

*Tidiness*, "nearly a key term" in Brisbane and clearly manifested in the "Foucauldian holy ground" that is the Royal Brisbane Hospital, is one of a number of possible names for the danger of personal and perhaps social obliteration that Michaels understands to threaten him: *homophobia, discrimination, bureaucracy*, would be one series of alternative names; *complacency, indifference, dismissal*, another. But *tidiness* has the advantage of getting at the centrality of a certain coercive requirement of homogeneity, conformity, and order, something like what David Wojnarowicz, for his part, castigated as the "pre-invented world" and the "one tribe nation," founded on fear of diversity. And *tidiness* also demonstrates the peculiarly hypocritical structure of the ordering requirement, so that Michaels's position paper is led to take the classically theoretical (or critical) path of showing that, in tidiness, things are not as they seem. Indeed, it demonstrates that suspicion is justified, because their apparent benignity masks actual hostility.

The hospital provides the perfect illustration of this. For what an AIDS patient needs, for survival, is a clean, germ-free environment, consonant with the PWA's high degree of vulnerability to infection, but what he encounters is a tidy one, the function of which is to "obscure dirt" (40/15). The floors are kept polished, and the top of the mobile table over Michaels's bed is cleaned twice a day: these are the surfaces, as Michaels points out, that the doctors and nurses see, and it is their perspective that defines the forms of orderliness that prevail in the institution. Meanwhile, however, the patient is exposed to grime that gathers on the ceiling, and "the underside [of the table], with which I actually come into contact, hasn't been swabbed since 1942 as far as I can judge" (43/17). To place a man with AIDS in an infectious diseases ward corresponds similarly to a logic of tidiness that for the patient is potentially lethal. And the only form of resistance that is possible in the face of such practices consists of not submitting passively to being tidied away by the hospital's coercive discipline. That is, it consists of practices of noncompliance: writing a critical diary, for example, and everything that for Michaels goes under the category of "working" but also something as apparently childish as keeping the TV badly tuned, on the grounds that it is a major instrument for inducing passivity. But noncompliance is also, and especially, everything we have already seen under the categories of lamentation and paranoia: complaining, criticizing, kvetching, and the deployment of sarcasm, until it "flood[s] the room and [sweeps] the entire nursing staff into the hall" (129/87).

Michaels's position paper, in other words, is the difficult patient's manifesto: it lays out why it is necessary for the AIDS patient, as part of the stage management of his dying, to do everything within his power to earn and maintain a place "at the top of the difficult patient list" (147/100). And, the hospital being emblematic of society at large, it shows also why the same response must be extended, beyond the hospital staff and the "lackeys" of the Immigration Department, to the full range of "specificities" that are lined up against you: the grubby landlord and the dishonest carpet cleaning company, the neighbors who play the wrong music and play it loudly or who block access to the Hill's Hoist, but also new university colleagues and—most particularly, perhaps—old friends to the extent that they prove (as prove they must by difficult patient logic) inconsiderate or unempathetic or just plain irritating. If the complaining passage I quoted earlier is a good example of such "difficult patient" peevishness, the diary as a whole is an extended record of Michaels's success in keeping up this taxing performance—this "art of being difficult," to adapt Malcolm Bowie's phrase in reference to Mallarmé—to the end.

It is worth pausing, though, to reflect briefly on the way this difficult patient performance also, like Michaels's testamentary anxieties, is overdetermined by gayness. Being difficult, we know, is an option that forms part of an alternative, between stage-managing the PWA's dying and survival and just giving up and going (139/94): submission and passivity as a form of suicide. But, if the temptation to give in is recognized as a manifestation of internalized homophobia, then tidiness theory, and the behaviors it authorizes (being difficult and the cultivation of paranoia), can be seen as reactions that function to obscure and displace a deep vulnerability on Michaels's part, his personal vulnerability to homophobic assessments of his value as an individual and the disease as a phenomenon. "How have I allowed myself to internalize this guilty attitude which makes me apologize for being ill, and promise to go quietly?" Michaels asks rhetorically (76/41) after an interview with his dean, having a little earlier described himself, "ashamed and cowering" (71/37) at the beach, although wanting to jump in for a swim. Two weeks later he seeks professional help because he feels "suicidal and crazy" (78/42). The visibility of KS lesions is part of the issue here, of course, as it is in *Silverlake Life:* "I can't manage my flawed countenance, and know it's only going to get worse" (80/44); "It's getting more and more difficult to look in the mirror" (87/49); "I turn myself off" (96/55)—until finally, under the relatively cheering stimulus of a trip to Sydney, he simply decides that "if my appearance bothered others, it should remain their problem" (106/62).

Beyond the anxiety about KS in this sequence, though, a more fundamental insecurity is suggested by Michaels's interesting analysis of the fragility of gay identity and of the role of desire and of sexual "promiscuity" in reinforcing it. The "enforced celibacy" of AIDS, he concludes (generalizing from his own experience, since AIDS does not in and of itself enforce celibacy, although it may on occasion diminish desire), is therefore a threat to gay men's sense of self: "If psychologists are right about the centrality and the fixity of identity for the human self, what terrible psychic violence something like AIDS must wreak on gays—and has perhaps done to me" (100/58). The psychologism of this passage is surprising, on the part of one who declares himself more indebted intellectually to Zen than to Freud and expresses elsewhere his suspicion of psychological explanations: it suggests a moment of introspection, here, that reverses the paranoid insistence on the important social forces at stake in personal experience and acknowledges, instead, the individual pain inflicted by social attitudes. Thus, on the occasion of an early hospital visit Michaels had written, with feeling: "Mama, you wouldn't believe how people treat you here. It's not the rubber gloves, or face masks, or bizarre plastic wrapping around everything. It's the way people address you, by gesture, by eye, by mouth" (25/4). Of course, in fact it

## Anxious Reading

is both of these, and especially the relation between the two. But passages like these force the conclusion that the difficult patient persona is not the product of some deficiency in Eric Michaels's character. Rather, it is a polemically constructed response directed externally to "the way people address you, by gesture, by eye, by mouth," and masking to some extent the degree to which it functions to bolster also an internally fragile, and internally threatened, sense of identity, damaged by its own internalization of those alienating gestures, looks, and words.

That the way people address you implies a polemical counter-address in the form of being difficult brings me, however, to a second aspect of the difficult patient performance, which is that, constituting a counter-address in the context of Michaels's dying, it also informs the structures of textual address in his writing, as a tactics of survival. If the diary's insistence on a generic status similar to that of a will and a position paper has to do with eluding the perceived danger of its obliteration by Warlpiri mourning customs and/or the forces of tidiness, the adaptation of the complex rhetoric of being difficult to the writing of the journal is part of a very carefully judged project designed to ensure that, having escaped obliteration, *Unbecoming* will go on to enjoy a posthumous afterlife by finding a readership. Being difficult is essential, in other words, both to the stage management of Michaels's dying (in which it protects a vulnerable identity) and to the stage management of his posthumous afterlife (in which it protects a social project), and in this latter respect the diary contains evidence of very careful thought regarding both the tactics of address (a stylistic matter) and the politics of publication (a pragmatic one) that will ensure such an afterlife.

Michaels understands, for example, that his obscurity as a public figure does not permit his writing to command the mass audience that Paul Foss seems to consider possible. But, given his notoriety among the Sydney intelligentsia (roughly equivalent, as he amusingly puts it, to the subscription list of *Art & Text*), he might hope for what he calls a "cult" following. And it happens (given the politics of oppositionality) that "these may be just the folks I wanted to talk to" (153/104): those that the diary *can* reach are, by a fortunate dispensation, also its ideal audience, the readers who can be expected to be responsive to it. This, in turn, means that a provocative tactics of address, an unbecoming rhetoric equivalent to the performance of being a difficult patient, although it would alienate a mass audience, might well be appropriate for a text signed by Eric Michaels. The opposite of Guibert's soft-pedal approach is in order.

> I think now I've escaped the worst of the possible consequences of being discovered (so longed for in my youthful quest for stardom), so that even if Paul is right that these diaries can get a wider than cult reading, no worries mate! And that's why Juan can paint the cover and I can call the thing *Unbecoming* (though I still like *Should Have Been a Dyke*). (153/104)

The thought here is condensed and allusive, but it unpacks fairly readily. The audience that a "star" might reach (imagine if Rock Hudson had left an AIDS diary) would inhibit a set of rhetorical practices—indicated by the title *Unbecoming* and the plan to have the provocative artist Juan Davila do a cover portrait—that are those to which Michaels is in any case drawn. Whatever the actual readership may prove to be in the end, an unbecoming address to a cult following is initially well calculated and strategic. So, no worries: "I have the satisfaction, my anger transsubstantiated" (153/104).

What this restriction of audience means in practice is that to our embryonic list of generic models for the diary (the will and the position paper) can now be added the posthumous revenge letter, as a vehicle simultaneously for the "transsubstantiation" of the author's anger and for the recruitment of an interested (Michaels's word will be *engaged*) readership. The revenge letter is a strikingly effective means of carrying on, beyond one's death, the performance of being a difficult patient, that is, of resisting victimhood by not taking it lying down. And *Unbecoming* includes (*en abyme*, as it were) three gems of the genre (66–70/34–37), addressed respectively to the sleazy landlord, an inconsiderate friend, and the offending carpet cleaning company. It also includes an example of "revenge publication," reproducing *in extenso* the hypocritical and self-contradictory (tidying) letter Michaels received, a month before his death, from the Immigration Department announcing that he would be deported ("to nowhere") as soon as he was medically fit to travel. One imagines the glee with which these letters were composed or transcribed into the diary for later publication.[1]

But, in addition to the "satisfaction" it affords the preposthumous author, the posthumously published revenge letter, as a denunciation of the inadequacies that have hastened a dying man to his grave, makes an irresistible appeal also to a certain kind of readership. It turns the knife in the wound of survivor guilt, whether the actual guilt of those who recognize themselves in the book or the vicarious guilt of those able to recognize themselves in or identify with those the book pillories. And it appeals to the curiosity and *Schadenfreude* of those who enjoy watching others squirm or who squirm at taking pleasure in the spectacle of others' squirming. Those two, not mutually exclusive, categories could add up to a good number of people, of course. But equally significant is the fact that reading itself is generically positioned, in the revenge letter mode, as an act of survivorhood and as one that entails reflection on the theme of one's responsibility toward the now deceased author. If it is "the specificities that get us in the end" (156/106), the deficiencies of one's behavior toward the author—whether they consist of dubious business practices or of inconveniently borrowing and keeping a VCR or of being the reader of a text whose availability to the public is predicated on the author's death (let alone getting some form of pleasure out of it)—are necessarily tinged with culpability. And it is, of course, definitionally, the effect of a difficult patient performance to define caregiving, whether pre- or, as in the case of the reader, postmortem, as inevitably deficient.

Such an intimately *involved* audience is what I understand Michaels to have in mind when he speaks of a "cult" following as being appropriate for *Unbecoming*, and it is as if he plans, therefore, to continue and extend, in the relation between his accusatory writing and its readers, the fraught relation with his actual friends that is compellingly described and analyzed—sometimes with affection, self-deprecation, and humor; sometimes more cantankerously—at a number of points in the volume (notably 43–44/18, 48–49/21–22, 126/85, 150/101–2). As *Silverlake Life* already suggested, this positioning of readers (or viewers) as surviving "friends" might be thought

---

1. This is true from a reader's perspective, even though in fact, as Paul Foss (pers. comm., Dec. 5, 1995) informs me, the Immigration Department letter was inserted editorially into the text.

characteristic of the AIDS diary, as an adaptation of the personal genre of the private journal to the requirements of public witnessing. But, whereas *Silverlake* thinks in terms of the production of a loving community, it seems probable that Michaels was guided, on the one hand, by a disenchanted estimate of the intelligentsia's motivation for reading and, on the other, by his perception of "the scale of Australian demography" (61/31), in which members of the academy, of the worlds of media and the arts, the bureaucracy, and political culture all seem to know one another and indeed to be closely, if not intimately, interconnected: in other words, they form an extended gossip circle. This unsentimental approach to the problem of readership leads him to rely, in other words, on word-of-mouth, at least in the first instance, placing his faith in some of the more unsavory motivations humans may have for reading a book and looking for a *succès de scandale* and a *succès de curiosité* in order to get his volume launched (this is stage management as one of the fine arts). But it also, and in the long run more significantly, tends to define the *kind* of reading (guilty, anxious, involved, "close to") that is required by the continuation, in book form, of the performance of Michaels the difficult patient.

As the hospital staff and Michaels's friends were put in a double bind by a patient who both needs their care and is never satisfied with it, so the reader of *Unbecoming*, as the addressee of a symbolic revenge letter, is interpellated in a way that is calculated to produce anxiety and guilt. Where writerly paranoia derives from the perception that vital social forces are implicated in the circumstances of an individual life, the culpability that can come to be associated with the act of reading has to do with the social responsibility a supposedly personal and private act may incur and, more specifically, in this and in similar cases, with the responsibility for survival—the survival of an oppositional spirit—that is entrusted to one's readerly status as survivor. But a survivor, notably in the kind of dire circumstances that call for witnessing, is always to some degree open to the suspicion (even if it is only anxious self-questioning) of having in some sense collaborated with the forces that make victims of others. Readerly status thus allies one, to all intents and purposes, with the prevailing forces of order and tidiness rather than with oppositionality. In that sense one is the addressee of a Lacanian demand that one is not in a position to fulfill, a demand that by definition *cannot* be fulfilled, and such a demand is calculated, therefore—because it is an appeal that comes framed as an accusation (something like: "Why don't you save me?")—to make reading an experience of disquiet, inadequacy, and anxiety.

This effort to destabilize the reader's equanimity and to produce anxiety in its place by making the unbecoming of the body the occasion of an unbecoming rhetorical performance is already visible in an astonishing predictive image that the reader encounters before even embarking on the text. It is simultaneously a frontispiece and the book's photographic *mise en abyme*; it is also one of the most remarkable representations of the AIDS body known to me; and, finally, like the text itself, it stages a compelling continuity between unbecoming's two, preposthumous and posthumous, stages. It is the product of a photography session, reported in the diary, that took place two months before the author's death, one of a series of "shots that might serve as graphics if needed. [. . .] All nude to the waist down [sic], featuring the cancer lesions most prominently" (152/103). It has been taken with a flash, so that certain physical details are highlighted, but in the first instance it is the subject's posture that is most striking, divided between a relaxed and seemingly passive torso (not noticeably thin but spotted with lesions) and an astoundingly alive face and head with luxuriant hair and beard, intense eyes, and— the *punctum* as well as the *studium* (Barthes)—a mouth open so that KS lesions can also be seen on the protruding tongue. In its own fashion this image thus stages the tension readable in the text, between the temptation of passiveness and the necessity of fierce resistance— the tension that makes this gesture of defiantly showing the body's state of unbecoming, "featuring the cancer lesions most prominently" (the photo's raison d'être), the mark of a signal victory over submission to the coercive conventions of tidiness and over Michaels's own complicitous willingness to give up and just go.

But the focal point is the tongue, its flesh catching the light and the lesions visible, a tongue that, given the intensity of expression in the face and eyes (will? defiance? rage?) can be seen, in addition to displaying the ravages of cancer, to be unmistakably performing the gesture of impertinence known (in schoolyards and elsewhere) as "sticking out one's tongue"—a singularly unbecoming gesture, its childishness (in an adult) suggestive of impotence, perhaps, but with

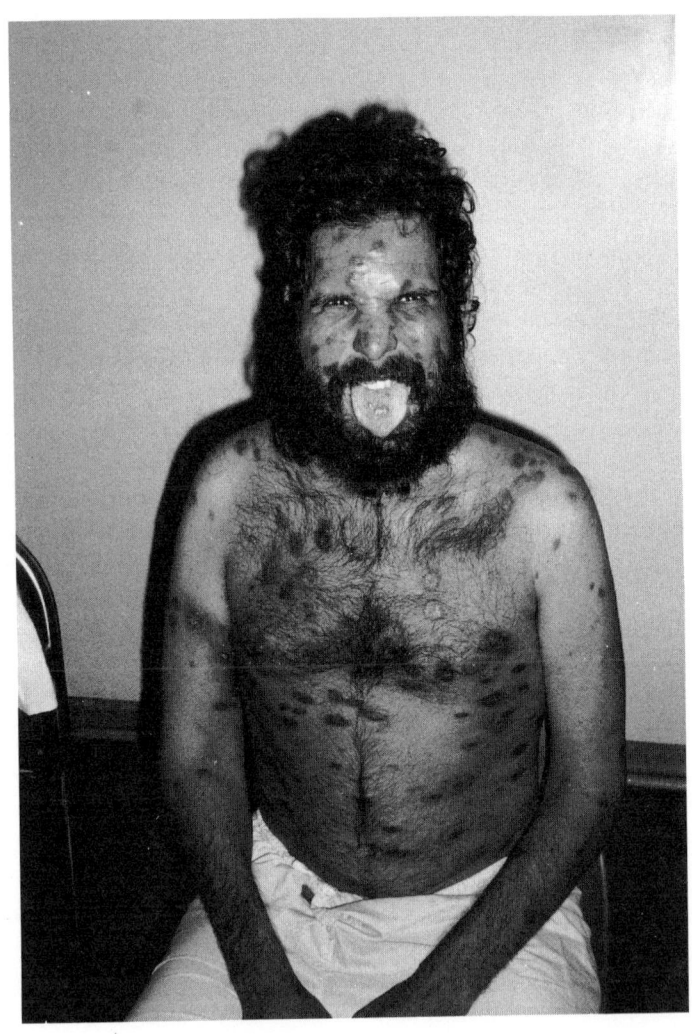

Fig. 1. Eric Michaels, Brisbane, June 26, 1988. (Photo by Penny Taylor.)

## Anxious Reading

implications of defiance and revenge as well as accusation and anger. These flash shots were intended as aids to Juan Davila's work on the portrait planned for the cover (which, in the end, this photo replaces), and this photo clearly makes ironic reference to the erotic motif of the protruding tongue in Davila's own work.[2] But the intended front-cover positioning makes it clear, if such corroborating evidence is necessary, that the gesture of impertinence is directed, into the photo's future, at us: the survivors of Michaels's death, the viewers of the photo, and the readers of his text.

In addition to the book's effort to confront in this way the reader's presumed complacency, however, the extended tongue also figures, therefore, a certain mediatory desire: I mean the desire to bridge the space—the space of death—that separates the thin, two-dimensional plane of the photograph, in which the author is confined, from the three-dimensional world in which the viewer-reader lives and moves and, penetrating that space, to exert effective impact within the viewer's (survivor's) world. Poignant because it figures the picture's authority, then, and by extension that of Michaels's text, as an authority borrowed from death, the tongue also figures the power to disturb that the text thereby acquires, beyond the death of the owner of the tongue. For a tongue, qua tongue, stands, obviously enough, for language—but *this* tongue carries the "morphemes" of AIDS and is marked by disease, so the message it delivers can only concern its owner's unwilling and refractory encounter with, and resistance to, the death that gives the message its power.

It would be wrong to assume, though, that there is anything ghostly or wraithlike in the image presented by Michaels's body. If the protruding tongue is accusatory, it does not threaten to "haunt" the reader-survivor but, rather, to extend itself materially into the postmortem domain so as to pursue a continuing policy of defiance and destabilization, harassment and difficultness—a matter less of metaphysics than of rhetoric and politics. In the EMPress edition of *Unbecoming* there is a back-jacket photo of Michaels: film-star handsome, well groomed, with a clipped mustache and stylish clothes (presumably an ID picture: Eric Michaels just off the plane in 1982?). This image is in striking and significant contrast with the frontispiece photo: the wild hair, the bushy beard, the fierce eyes, the

---

2. See his "Beauty and the Beast" (1982), "The Kiss" (1982), "ARt I$ H̶o̶m̶o̶s̶e̶x̶-̶u̶a̶l̶" (1983), and especially "The Studio" (1984), reproduced in Taylor.

determined expression, the body invaded by lesions, the extended tongue and its aggressive gesture. In this adult face, with its wild features, the tongue seems to allude to a famous feature of Polynesian iconography—familiar to many from the Maori "haka" performed by New Zealand teams before football games—in which a protruding tongue signifies warlike ferocity. But, more generally, the contrast with the jacket photo makes this an image of Michaels as *wild man*, that is, as a social persona (more than an individual) and as a figure who lives on the edge—or beyond the pale—of orderly, civilized society and harasses it with a kind of guerilla warfare, even if his mission is only to offer a critical counterimage that refuses to be tidied away or otherwise to disappear. This portrait of the author as wild man is thus the sign of *Unbecoming*'s own mission of harassment, its ambition to function as the permanent thorn in the side of Tidy Town and the continuing Foucauldian horror show. And in this respect we might also be led to think, therefore, and again in terms of social place and function rather than of individual identity, of the aboriginality to which the image also, unmistakably, makes iconographic reference.

I'm not claiming that in *Unbecoming* Michaels is producing AIDS as a way for white people to achieve the political status of Aboriginal people. That would be sentimental, and, more to the point, it would be insensitively exploitative of the shameful two-hundred-year history of Aboriginal contact with, and resistance to, the genocidal white settlement of Australia. But there is a certain structural homology between the difficult historical survival of aboriginality and the resistance to murderous tidiness, the struggle against the horror show, that Michaels posits—it is a "first principle"—as necessary. And the five or six years I assume to separate the trim Eric Michaels of the jacket photo and the "wild man" AIDS image of *Unbecoming* correspond, for Michaels, to the Yuendumu years, in the course of which—without being or imagining himself to be a Warlpiri Aboriginal—he earned an identity and a place among the Warlpiri people, who were engaged in an inspired, if wild (unauthorized, extralegal, *sauvage*), communicational practice of their own: an appropriation of, and so an effective intervention in, the technology, structure, and apparatus of contemporary televisual culture.

They invented and operated a collectively run TV station, maneuvering in this way, from the margins, as a matter of self-defense and in their own interests: defending their culture from the destructive incursions of modernity while simultaneously giving it a "voice" within the culture of modernity and ensuring therefore what Michaels (1994) significantly—and, in the context of *Unbecoming*, poignantly—called a cultural future. These years are referred to in the diary (124/84) as the Birth of a Station, and it is possible to think that the Warlpiri example furnished another general model—alongside the position paper, the will, and the revenge letter but (like the protruding tongue) more pragmatic than generic—for the rhetorical operation being performed in *Unbecoming*. This could be described as the birth of a "status," posthumous but effective, and hence the achievement of a cultural future, for an untidy, marginalized, wild subject whose body will die of AIDS.

If Michaels is careful, then, at the diary's outset to deny any claim to an Aboriginal identity, he is led toward the end to include, symmetrically, a thoughtfully worded statement of the reasons that underlie his affection for and affinity with Aboriginal people:

> they are engaged, in a way that white Australians tend not to be. Their circumstances are interesting, to them and me. They tend to be kind. And no matter how hard they try, they mostly fail to be bourgeois. They are too familiar with poverty and suffering, perhaps. I feel a whole lot less self-conscious about the way I look and my visible marks of disease when I'm with blacks. They seem a good deal less concerned. (124–25/84)

But here he is obviously not referring to a model of rhetorical effectiveness so much as he is defining a preferred mode of reception, for his own diseased self and so, by extension, for *Unbecoming*. Aboriginality is not the identity Michaels claims for himself so much as it names a certain like-mindedness and capacity for "kindness," a failure to be bourgeois that guarantees the kind of understanding—not "concern" but "engagement"—that *Unbecoming* as a rhetorical performance would like to encounter.

The terminological distinction that frames the whole passage may seem subtle, though, and the text offers no definitions. The gloss I would offer introduces the concept of "involvement" as a mediating term. To be concerned, as, in Michaels's experience, white Australians tend to be, faced with the writing of AIDS on his face, is to be interested and even sympathetic but without being involved (and, so, unempathetic). Perhaps indeed one can go so far as to say that concern is a way of disengaging oneself and one's responsibility, but without seeming to, according to a duplicitous structure that would align concern with tidiness (which pretends, for example, to be "concerned" with health when it is actually devoted to the preservation of a certain kind of order). The health minister mentioned in *Unbecoming* who—"sympathetics" notwithstanding—reassured his audience that "we (gays, IV drug users, hemophiliacs) are not members of the 'general public'" (181/123) was demonstrating concern (as politicians often do) while simultaneously withholding empathy and tidying AIDS out of sight (and so, for his viewers, out of mind as well) by means of a spurious exercise in categorization. Concern, then, is bourgeois because it is hegemonic, and it is a front for complacency and indifference.

Engagement, on the other hand, necessarily entails involvement, and in Michaels's usage it seems to refer more specifically to a combination of involvement—as something akin to the phenomenological concept of "thrownness" (*Geworfenheit*): finding oneself caught up, willy-nilly, in a situation—with a degree of disempowerment that prevents one from exerting control over it. *Resistance* is thus a synonym for *engagement*, in the cases in which resistance (in Certeau's handy metaphor) is obliged to be more tactical than strategic. Engagement defines oppositional practices that are untidy, then, like the Warlpiri invention of TV or the practice of noncompliance, the art of being difficult, that Michaels invents as a response to AIDS and the whole social horror show that goes with it—an art that extends to the rhetoric of *Unbecoming*. It is an anti-concern, and, because it corresponds to the practices of those whose "circumstances are interesting," it might be thought to be in the same relation to anxiety that concern is to complacency.

Engagement, then, by this definition, is a quality that it would be difficult for those in positions of power to achieve. It is engaged readers (on the "Aboriginal" model) that the diary seeks: they would be understanding of, and empathetic with, the embattled situation out of which Michaels speaks. But it is a concerned readership (on the "white" model) that it is most likely to reach, for historical reasons (having to do with the composition of the reading public in Australia and elsewhere) as well as for structural reasons (having to do with the power of readers, as survivors, with respect to a text's attempted survival). It is therefore a concerned readership, not one that can be assumed automatically to be engaged, that becomes the prime textual addressee in the diary. And the problem of address as a rhetorical proposition becomes that of converting readerly concern into something more like engagement—which, in the first instance, means *getting through* to concerned readers, penetrating the barrier of their disengagement, getting them involved in spite of themselves, and this across the space of death that makes the text's survival so crucially dependent on the involvement of these uninvolved survivors. Whence Michaels's worry over the "etiquette or sense of style [that] needs to be considered when agreeing to any, assumedly posthumous project" (144). Whence his calculus of scandal and curiosity, of gossip, as a way of engaging an audience. Whence finally his tactics of the protruding tongue, which sums up a whole difficult patient performance but also signifies a desire to break down the distance between Michaels and his posthumous audience, the text and its reception, and to pass on a certain "contamination"—not the infection of AIDS but the rhetorical transmission of a certain capacity for anxiety.

To expect engagement of an audience definitionally capable only of concern is, of course, asking for more than that audience can give: it is a recipe for producing a double bind structured like a Lacanian demand. This is never truer than in the case of an audience of readers, since, except in its most mechanical sense, reading is a phenomenon that presupposes distance with respect to a text. As opposed to supposedly "direct" communication, reading enacts effects of difference and deferral in the communication process and entails arts of exegesis and interpretation. If by "involvement" in a text is meant either the capacity for a fully absorbed attention or (what is in the final analysis the same thing) the capacity fully to realize its apparently limitless effects of signification, reading falls short of that degree of involvement. Its response being a specifically mediated and so a differentially positioned (not to say conditioned) one, it falls short of the limitless demand made on it by a textuality that is itself defined by the death of the author, in the sense of an absence of any control over the range of its possible meanings.

The option available to a reader, then, is not so much between concern and engagement as it is between complacency and anxiety, that is, between an unselfconscious tidying away, through (facile) categorization and (reductive) interpretation, and a capacity for scruple in the face of the double bind in which one is placed. A concerned but scrupulous reader can make a genuine effort in the direction of involvement and engagement, but—this mechanism is relentless—the more scrupulous the effort, the less easy it becomes to be sure that one has escaped mere concern. And, conversely, the more unselfconscious the concern, the more easily it can mistake itself for engagement. The alternative to concern, then, for a reader caught in the problematics of distance that readerly difference implies is not engagement but anxiety. Anxiety is what arises, for a scrupulous reader, from the fact of being separated from direct textual access by the author's death, which itself grounds the act of reading, whether that phrase be understood in a theoretical or an actual sense, so that the double bind the distance of reading enforces is similar in its effect to the double bind inflicted on the friends and caregivers of a difficult patient: the more they try, the less they succeed.

There is, in short, no escaping the fact—it's a given, a first principle, if not a matter of *Geworfenheit*—that reading entails power and that a text is relatively disempowered (by its author's "death" or death) with respect to its reading, which means, on the one hand, that readerly engagement is definitionally excluded (if engagement entails disempowerment) and, on the other, that the best-intentioned reader is necessarily drawn in the direction of the hegemonic, enforcing norms and conventions, by way of tidying up and containing the manifestations of textual disorderliness. Reading, as Michel de Certeau might put it, is inevitably more strategic than it is tactical.[3] Such is the nature of what is called "interpretation"—and in critical circles something called "strong reading" is often particularly appreciated. "Weak reading," though, if one were to try to imagine it—a *lettura debole* along the lines of Gianni Vattimo's *pensiero debole?*—would not be closer to the ideal of engagement, because it would be merely compliant. It would reverse the text/reader power structure rather

---

3. I am not forgetting that Certeau himself describes "reading as poaching" as tactical. But he is working here with a model of text as the cultural "given" that individuals have to learn to "inhabit," like moving into a rented apartment or "walking in the city." This is a conception of text that has no space for the death of the author, although it is of course that death, in its theoretical sense, that makes readerly poaching possible.

than producing the encounter, on the plane of oppositionality—an encounter of mutual engagements—of which Michaels seems to dream.

Engaged reading, then, in its ideal form, is a utopia. The best a militantly uncompliant text like *Unbecoming* can achieve, although it is somewhat less than it demands, is the sort of anxiously involved reading I described as scrupulous, a reading that is uncertain of itself because it is conscious, however hard it tries, of its own failure to be anything but concerned. This is a way of failing that is at the opposite pole from the ease with which Aboriginals, as described by Michaels, fail to be bourgeois (it's a failure, equally easy, not to be bourgeois, if you will). But it does have something in common, perhaps—a certain desperate vigilance, for instance—with the unremitting effort of the difficult patient to resist and to go on resisting, despite the temptation to give in, to become passive, to go under, to disappear. A well-grounded fear of complacency, on one side, responds to a well-grounded fear of compliance, on the other. The dying author's extended tongue, then (which, after all, corresponds to a compliant medical gesture as well as being an act of defiance), teaches us, perhaps, that as readers we *can* get some way out of our concern and into an area of anxiety, and it is in that area of anxiety that maybe, just maybe, it might be possible to meet the tongue halfway.

6

## *RSVP*, or Reading and Mourning

> "What are you doing next, Mr. Jarman?" After, after, after,
> that's the problem when you survive.
> —JARMAN

If you go back to the influential essay by Barthes that launched the phrase "the death of the author," it is immediately clear that Barthes was concerned not with a problem of survival (and continuity) but with a project of substitution and, so, of discontinuity. The famous final clause—"the birth of the reader must be at the cost of the death of the Author" (Barthes 1977, 148)—sounds almost callous, therefore. But this is because, for Barthes, the figures of the author and the reader are standing in for different orders of discourse that, in a somewhat polemical way, are being starkly opposed: the Author (with a capital *A*) stands for an ideology of communication in which agents are at least partly autonomous, and the Author's opposite number is not the reader, therefore, but the Critic (we are being referred to Barthes's polemic in the 1960s against "University criticism" and in favor of the French *nouvelle critique*). The reader, on the other hand, who goes uncapitalized, refers us to a concept of writerliness, or textuality, that is described in this essay as "originless" (its "scriptor" is not the origin of text) because it is a function of language itself. This is the reader whose *jouissance* (bliss) will later be described in *Le plaisir du texte*. The writer and the reader, for Barthes, are not persons but mere functions of language, whose personal agency is incidental, as it were, to their function in a liberated, expansive economy of writing and reading.

But, if the Author and the Critic are allegorical figures, as their capital letters seem to indicate, the uncapitalized reader and writer (or scriptor) are themselves purely mythic, in the sense that they are conceived by Barthes only in the context of a language completely disengaged from effects of discourse (where *discourse* refers to the set of all systems of signification and corresponding signifying practices, together with the relations, whether of subjectivity or of personality, that are produced as an effect of these systems and practices). If the Author and the Critic enjoy autonomous status and agency with respect to language, the writer and the reader are agents of a writerliness and a readerliness that are imagined and that we are asked to imagine, in turn, as purely linguistic effects independent of the order of discourse. "A pure gesture of inscription (and not of expression)" is Barthes's phrase for the action of writing, and the gesture traces a "field without origin" (1977, 146) because he is already, in anticipation of his work in the 1970s, attempting to conceive of writing as an "intransitive" operation that would be "ideology" free, as opposed to "transitive" or functional (communicative) *uses* of language—that is, discourse. Never mind that language never occurs independently of discursive effects; the reader whose "birth" is celebrated in "La mort de l'auteur" ("The Death of the Author") is an entirely theoretical incarnation of this (desire for an) "intransitive" function of language. And the Author (but consequently "the author" as well) can therefore be allowed by Barthes to disappear from the scene of theoretical speculation unregretted.

The substitutions Barthes is effecting in his essay are, of course, polemical in intent, and so they constitute the essay itself as a fine example not of the intransitivity it desires but of linguistic transitivity as a discursive phenomenon. Witnessing, too, is a polemical action, but it is a discursive act to which surviving, not substitution, is crucial, precisely to the extent that surviving is a response to the desire on the part of some to bring about substitutions, that is, to cause certain "figures" (read: persons) to disappear so that they may be replaced by others, in the way that Barthes "disappears" the Author to the benefit of the reader. Reading, from the point of view of witnessing, is thus a site not of substitution but of survival and one to which the death of the author (with a small *a*) cannot ever be a matter of complete indifference, therefore, precisely because such indifference would imply on the reader's part a relation of substitution, not of continuity, with respect to the author. But the death of the author, in the sense of a loss of authorial control over signification, is nevertheless the condition of possibility of reading, so that survival-through-reading cannot be conceived as a matter of pure, undiluted

## RSVP, or Reading and Mourning

continuity: it is definitionally subject not to the interruption that would substitute reader for author but to a real degree of discontinuity within the continuity it produces.

Living to tell the tale (surviving to write so as to be read) is, of course, a constant theme in witnessing literature, and one might say, using Barthes's verb, that a witnessing subject is born whenever a potential victim, in conditions of extreme duress, foresees the possibility, remote as it may be, of becoming a narrator: the narrator of the events that themselves seem likely to reduce the witness to silence. AIDS writing honors this urge to live to tell the tale in many narrative, dramatic, filmic, and poetic accounts of the epidemic and its effects, and AIDS diaries respond to it also to the extent that they represent an option, on the part of the author, not to die immediately (by suicide) but to stay alive in order to write. But an AIDS diarist is also, one might say, dying to tell the tale not only in the sense that the story the writer is anxious to narrate ("dying to tell") is itself a story of survival—of living on in order to write—but also because the author's dying is a way of making the story "telling." Its living on is predicated on its protagonist's death as an author, and on the writing of that story of authorial dying, as a condition of survival through the form of (dis)continuity that is reading. The AIDS diarist does not "survive to write in order to be read," then, so much as the story's survival is itself predicated on the reading that his option in favor of writing implies as its indispensable complement. Because the diarist does not foresee living to become a narrator so much as an authorial decision to live in order to write itself foresees the survival of a subject of textuality, the responsiveness of the reader, the guarantee of a certain relation of continuity as opposed to the absolute discontinuity of indifference and substitution, becomes a matter of primary concern. For one cannot bear witness to one's own death (the statement "I am dead" cannot be uttered) except by recourse to representation and, hence, to the reading through which the *énoncé* "I am dying" can come to signify "'I' is dead."

But survival then, whether in the form of living to tell the tale or of dying to tell it, is synonymous with *deferral*, and acts of witness are necessarily acts of deferred (not "immediate" or "direct") communication. A narrator who survives to tell the tale is no longer the potential victim whose initial access to witnessing lay in the desire to survive so that the story might be told; that desire was, indeed, a first displacement with respect to absolute victimhood that doubles for the event of survival itself, a prolepsis of the survival that makes the narrative a deferred act (it will be written in the past tense). A fortiori, the author whose project of witnessing lay in the urge to die in such a way that the story of his dying could be told—that is, by writing—survives only by virtue of the relay furnished by the writing and by the reading that makes the writing signify: not the event of survival, in this case, but the event of death intervenes, even though the initial option to live and to write defined witnessing as a function of survival (of survival so as to die writing). Here, then, the fact of deferred communication becomes the very sign of the death to which the communication bears witness at the same time as it is the vehicle through which survival becomes possible.

That is why it puts reading in what might be called a "stressed" (not to say distressed) position: stressed in the sense of emphasized, because stress falls on the responsibility enjoined on the reader—the responsibility to be responsive, if I may play on the common etymology of these two words (from *spondere*, "to say yes")—but stressed, too, in the sense of anxious, because the responsibility of responsiveness is necessarily exercised under conditions of deferral that make the value, and indeed the possibility, of responsiveness dubious. The reader, one might say, is positioned as the "sponsor" (one who says yes) of the act of authorial witness, taking responsibility on behalf of, but also in lieu of, a supposedly "original" witness who was in fact (always) already displaced into representation and, having become irretrievable, can be said therefore *not to have survived*, even as the requirement that the witnessing be made to survive subsists.

The stressed position AIDS diaries allocate to readership is one that is itself readable in the texts, as I have tried to indicate. Its clearest and most explicit statement, though, is in a remarkable passage from Dreuilhe's *Corps à corps:*

> Mon espoir inconscient est que ce livre, surgi comme une excroissance cancéreuse, hors de mon cerveau, devienne un appendice monstrueux qu'il sera possible de séparer finalement de mon corps. J'imagine que chaque phrase, chaque image de ce livre se substituera à un de mes lymphocites fauchés par le SIDA. Dans mon univers délirant, l'écriture n'est pas seulement une thérapie mais une pratique magique.

## RSVP, or Reading and Mourning

En tendant à l'épidémie le miroir de mon journal, je peux espérer décapiter le Gorgone sans qu'il me pétrifie. Le philtre dans lequel je plonge aussi mes angoisses et obsessions sera d'autant plus efficace que mon audience sera plus vaste. Chacun de mes lecteurs deviendrait un de mes soldats. Je rêve d'endoctriner, d'enrégimenter tous ceux qui me lisent, pour qu'ils me sauvent. Une fois le cordon ombilical coupé entre le livre et moi, je me serai peut être soulagé de mon SIDA, par cette conjuration de mots que j'essaie d'aligner dans l'ordre voulu. (178–79)

[My unconscious hope is that this book, emerging out of my brain like a cancerous excrescence, might become a monstrous appendix that it will finally be possible to separate from my body. I imagine that each sentence, each image in the book will substitute for one of my AIDS-demolished lymphocytes. In my delirious universe, writing is not just a therapy but a magical practice. By holding up the mirror of my diary to the epidemic, I can hope to cut off the Gorgon's head without being turned to stone. The potion in which I dip my anguish and obsessions also will be all the more efficacious as my audience will be large. Each of my readers would become one of my soldiers. I dream of indoctrinating all who read me, enrolling them under my banner, so that they will save me. Once the umbilical cord will have been cut between the book and myself, I will perhaps prove to have shucked off my AIDS, through this conspiracy of words that I am trying to line up in the requisite order.][1]

This passage merits lengthy exegesis, so closely does it reproduce—within Dreuilhe's characteristically military metaphorics—the structures of thought associated with "the writing of AIDS," as I have tried to delineate them in this essay: the writing of the body conceived as a transcription that will survive the body's death by reaching a readership willing to be "engaged" (enrolled, recruited, *enrégimenté*), in spite of the distance of death that is figured here, at the end, by the cutting of the umbilical cord and, at the beginning, by

---

1. I translate from the original French, Linda Coverdale's translation being a little too free for my purposes.

the image of the book as a cancerous excrescence that can be cut cleanly off the author's body. I will stress only two particular points, though. One, Dreuilhe's willingness to make explicit his "unconscious" hope that writing will function magically as a cure, conditioned on mixing the potion right and lining up the lymphocyte words in the requisite order, can certainly be assumed to lay bare an unacknowledged motivation of AIDS writing in general and of the AIDS diary in particular. The crazy, delirious hope is that "facing it" by means of representation, capturing "it"'s image—the image of AIDS, the image of death—in the mirror of writing will make it possible both, heroically, to decapitate the Gorgon and to survive, like Theseus, the fate of petrifaction. The mythic model is a powerful one. But, concomitantly (and this is my second point), the responsibility placed on Dreuilhe's reader is also made explicit and explicitly exorbitant: it is nothing less than to "save" the dying author, heroic as he may be in his own "write." The cure of the author is not only a function of the mirror held up Theseus-like to AIDS in his writing but also of the "indoctrination" of a readership that is required to be so engaged, so *totally* committed to the author's cause, that the Gorgon will prove powerless.

So strong is Dreuilhe's vision of salvation here that deferral, as such, is not an explicit issue (although it is, of course, implied by his emphasis on the mediations of writing and reading). On the other hand, so many elements in this passage—phrases like "unconscious hope" and "delirious universe," the deployment of verbs of imagining and dreaming, the prudent modalization of verbs through subjunctive forms, the appearance of the adverb *perhaps* and the careful phrase "je peux espérer" (I can hope)—insist on the author's knowledge that his desire for cure, his appeal to the reader to save him, are phantasmatic, if not frankly illusory, that what is finally transmitted to the reader is less the naked demand that reading effect the author's cure than the anxiety to which that demand responds, that is, the desire for such a cure to be possible associated with the knowledge that it is not. But, since the demand is nevertheless made, the reader is put in the classic double-bind situation of being made the addressee of an urgent appeal (save me) while learning simultaneously that the appeal is phantasmatic and that readers cannot do what is here, nevertheless, asked of them. Much as in the case of *Unbecoming*, what is most efficaciously transmitted, in the end, then, is anxiety—an anxiety that is, among other things, an anxiety about the effects of death on communication—so that it is the transmission of anxiety about the diminished prospects for survival that reading represents, that itself becomes the vehicle of authorial (textual) survival. And reading that wishes to be responsive to the appeal for cure made by the text is necessarily stressed, therefore, by the knowledge it shares with the text, that such responsiveness is always already rendered inadequate by the fact of death—the fact that is itself made concrete in the deferral of communication without which reading would be neither necessary nor (in anything other than a purely mechanical sense) possible.

There is a short film by the Canadian filmmaker Laurie Lynd that provides an opportunity, although it is not in diary form and does not specifically thematize reading, to reflect on the relation between what I have called stressed reading and the film's own explicit concern, which has to do with the nature of mourning and, less explicitly, with connections between mourning and witnessing. The film is entitled *RSVP*, and where it relates mourning and witnessing to a thematics of loss, it understands them more particularly in terms of a dynamics of authority that identifies a problematics of responsiveness as the effect—we can call it the survival effect—of deferred communication. *RSVP* is thus a film about mourning and witnessing in the specific context of survivorhood, as the "after, after, after" of which Jarman speaks in my epigraph. If deferred messages have a particular authority (borrowed from death), it lies in their power to demand response, but, since response is always and inevitably inadequate, in the face of death's reality, that inadequacy implies that the task of responding is never done and must be relayed in turn and relayed, of course, endlessly.

The film is set in Toronto. A youngish man, Sid, enters an empty house, evidently just home from a trip. He reads a message taped to a mirror and releases the cat into the garden. The phone rings, but he does not answer it: we hear a jointly recorded message that enables us, although one may not realize it on a first viewing, to hear the "live" voice of Sid's recently deceased lover, Andy, who has died of AIDS and from whose funeral in Winnipeg Sid is returning. With the note on the mirror this is the first of many instances in the film of a deferred message made possible by the technology of representation (re-presentation), and, as the friend who is calling now records his message (a second instance), the support he offers makes the viewer realize Sid's state of bereftness. A glimpse of a hospital bed set up by the French windows looking out into the garden confirms the perception (never specifically confirmed) that AIDS is the culprit.

As Sid looks at two sets of family photos—his own with Andy; then, on the refrigerator, those of Andy's parents separately, of Sid and Andy separately, and finally of Sid and Andy with a young woman, who will prove to be Andy's sister (whose lesbianism is briefly suggested)—he prepares to make tea and switches on the radio, as lonesome people may do "for company." It is a Canadian Broadcasting Corporation (CBC) request program, "RSVP," and Sid is just in time to catch an announcer *responding* to the request of one Andrew Sheldon, who, having been unable to attend a recent recital by Jessye Norman, has asked to hear the soprano's recording of Berlioz's "Le spectre de la rose," from *Les nuits d'été*. As the orchestral introduction fills the air, Sid stands motionless, his face troubled, then hastens to record the music, fumbling badly with the equipment as he does so. Deferral upon deferral: Andy, one realizes, has made the request before his death, setting it up as a message from beyond the grave (we will see later that the lovers own the Jessye Norman recording in their own collection, so there is evidence of intention on Andy's part). The complicated mechanism of radio technology, but also the built-in delay of request and response, are being employed in the service of a certain project of survival on Andy's part.

But survival through deferral is also implied in multiple ways by the song itself: a poem by Gautier, set by Berlioz, recorded by Norman, broadcast by CBC in a chain of relays, its own theme is that of survival. With its last faint perfume a wilted rose speaks to the (presumably beautiful young) woman who wore it to the ball and was thus responsible for the rose's death, but it speaks lovingly of its contentment to find itself lying, as if entombed in alabaster, on its wearer's breast. Gautier is consciously and specifically ("Ci-gît une rose [Here lies a rose]") referring his poem to the conventions of epitaph, whereby the "soul" of a deceased person speaks a message addressed to the living:

Ce léger parfum est mon âme,
Et j'arrive du paradis.

## RSVP, or *Reading and Mourning*

[This faint perfume is my soul,
And I come to you from paradise.]

But deferred, now, by the chain of relays, from its context of writing (in which it had the value, perhaps, of a piece of semi-bantering, over-precious, poetic wit), the poem of survival itself survives, albeit with a signification that in the new context is radically altered, since it has become a message from Andy and it speaks of AIDS, Gautier's ball becoming a possible reference to the good times associated with the urban gay lifestyle and the circumstances of the rose's death hinting at the possibility of Andy's having been infected by his lover. The authorial message (about roses and such) has "died" (although it persists from relay to relay as the poem's *énoncé*) in order for the poem to become readable as a text of AIDS witness. And the uncanny quality that derives from the "spectral" character of a message that survives, although so marked by death that its authority is profoundly altered (no longer a matter of bantering preciosity but something eerie and momentous), is of course reinforced by the music. Berlioz's orchestration is lush, luxurious, and often voluptuous but at times also hollow and mysterious, as if he were particularly sensitive to the connotations of death as the guest at life's feast that are in the poem. And the unearthly quality of Jessye Norman's operatically trained soprano voice, with its hint of sublimity and its own other-worldly quality (see Lyotard 1988, on "the inhuman"; and Frank 1995, on soprano voices), concretizes very powerfully the idea of a voice speaking "from paradise" with an authority derived from death.

As the music plays, the camera moves out from Sid's house to explore a community of friends (a lesbian and gay bookstore and counseling center with its bulletin board of obituaries to which Andy's is added) but also another environment: the high school where Andy taught and where the announcement of his death has been less lovingly vandalized with homophobic graffiti. When it returns, finally, to its point of departure and we discover Sid pacing the hallway as the haunting last measures, with their hollow woodwind orchestration, resound in the empty house:

> Ci-gît une rose
> Que tous les rois vont jalouser,

[Here lies a rose
That every king will envy,]

the context in which the message from beyond is received has consequently widened: it is no longer the house voided by AIDS but a social scene, one partly of warmth and companionship but also of hostility and confrontation. And, accordingly, the problem of family now enters the picture. Busying himself frantically with packing away Andy's things, Sid comes upon a sweater, draped over a chair at Andy's desk, as if he were still using it—the image has clear affinities with Guibert's similar thematization of the author's absent presence—and falls into contemplation. Then he goes to the phone and calls Ellen, Andy's sister in Winnipeg.

If the relays figure "Le spectre de la rose" as signifying the authority messages acquire through (death and) deferral, Ellen—as the (presumed) lesbian who is also "in touch" with the family—is the film's principal figure of mediation, that is, of relay, as a mode of continuity. Sid cannot communicate directly with Andy's parents, but Ellen is able to transmit to them his message about Andy's message of request and response, which, living in Winnipeg, they will be able to hear because the broadcast, in yet another instance of deferral, is time delayed. Her mother is responsive ("Of course I want to hear it. Thank you for telling me"), but it is also for her to retransmit Sid's message about Andy's message, this time to its final destination, Andy's father, the very figure, one supposes, of patriarchal authority in its homophobic incarnation. She does so by turning on the radio as she serves him his lunch. At first scowling and isolated behind his newspaper then troubled and moved, the father, as ultimate addressee of Andy's request for a response, remains—by contrast in particular with Ellen, who poignantly breaks down and gives way to grief as she stands listening to the music in her kitchen—not undisturbed but apparently unresponsive.

His response, when it comes, is thus delayed by a week. The film now, as it closes, echoes its opening scenes. As we see Sid approaching and entering his house again, we hear the answering machine once again speaking to the emptiness. Now only Sid's voice invites the caller to leave a message, but now, too, the caller is not a friend but Andy's father. "I just wanted to thank you for letting Ellen know about that song," he records. "I'm sorry we didn't get a chance to talk more at the funeral. We know what a big help you were to Andy. We know how important you were to him. Well, thanks." These, under the circumstances, are broken, poverty-stricken words, and they are not received directly by Sid (let alone by Andy, for whom they come too late); they are, so to speak, "under deferral." This deferred response to a much deferred message is clearly inadequate, and yet it is also something unhoped for, given the history of alienated affections the film allows us to guess at. For it *is* a response, and the implication is that this degree of (inadequate) responsiveness would not have been achieved had not Andy's message itself, by virtue of the authority it borrows from death (and deferral), had the particular power to elicit it. Nor would the message of Andy's witness have been efficacious had it not been retransmitted through a chain of witnessing relays embodied (leaving Gautier, Berlioz, Jessye Norman, and the CBC out of it, as the vehicles of the message) by Sid, as its first addressee, then by Ellen and her mother, as a series of "afters" that give it social impact, symbolically speaking, on top of its personal value to Sid. And, although the film achieves an effect of closure with the father's reception of and response to the message, one has to imagine also the further "broadcasting" of its own witnessing message, replicating Andy's, among the audiences who view it.[2] Consequently, this effect of broadcasting—of relay and retransmission, with all the effects of delay and deferral they imply—becomes finally the film's most encompassing metaphor for its understanding of what witnessing is and what witnessing entails.

But there is also mourning, and the sweater that, it will be remembered, provoked Sid's decision to retransmit to the family Andy's message, received and understood in the first instance by Sid as addressed to him. As the father records his message of apology, acknowledgment, and (perhaps) reconciliation, Sid again, as at the beginning, enters the house but this time removes his jacket, encountering as he does so the sweater that now hangs on the coatrack, the relic of Andy that signifies both his absence and the sense in which he

---

2. More accurately, *RSVP* presents chains of relays as the vehicle for acts of communication that are inserted in other chains of relays: thus, the chain Gautier-Berlioz-Norman-CBC mediates Andy's communication, across death, with Sid, and this communication initiates the chain that extends to Ellen, the mother and the father. It is then these two interlocking chains that form the vehicle of the film's communication with spectators, which opens the chain of which my account of *RSVP*, addressed to its own readership, forms part.

survives and remains present. At this point the memory stirs in Sid that gives the sweater its symbolic charge for him, one of those flashes of reminiscence, seemingly random, that mourners know well, and the film plays back the incident for us. Sid and Andy (whom we *see*, now, for the first and only time) are leaving the house together to attend a social engagement. To Sid's slight irritation Andy stops and returns to the house: he has forgotten the sweater. Sid: "It's not cold." Andy: "It's always cold in their house." Sid: "We'll be late." Andy: "We're always late." Andy quickly grabs the sweater off the rack, gives Sid an affectionate and reconciliatory peck, and they leave together.

This memory thus signifies that, if the sweater figures Andy's absent presence, what it means for the survivor, Sid, is a consciousness that it is nevertheless, in the "after"-life of his survivorhood, "always cold" and "always [too] late." The "after, after, after" of survivorhood (and witness) has, as its concomitant awareness, this sense of coldness and belatedness. Andy's sweater, of course, might keep Sid warm if he were able to break down the distance of his belatedness (the distance of death) and put it on: after all, he is wearing an undershirt that looks exactly similar to the one Andy is wearing in our brief glimpse of him (perhaps it is the same undershirt?). But we do not see him put it on: in the last shot of the movie he stands, staring and contemplative, by the coatrack. Who dares to think that they might step into a dead person's shoes or wear their sweater? The dead cannot survive, except figuratively, in us. What response would count as adequate to a message deferred by death? Our responses are always painfully insufficient because they necessarily always come too late, and that, for this film, is the meaning of mourning. All we can do—and this is the meaning of witness—is carry the message forward and pass it on, relay by relay, the closure that would signify an adequate response being endlessly deferred.

Andy's sweater, hanging forlornly on its rack, can thus symbolically articulate the twin themes I have wanted to develop in this essay: on the one hand, the *power* of representation, as deferred discourse borrowing its authority from death, with the potential for survival it offers; and, on the other, the inevitable *inadequacy* of a response to a deferred message, a response such as a reader might furnish, following the death of the author, and made therefore under circumstances of

## RSVP, or *Reading and Mourning*

survivorhood. Witnessing, as the desire to send the message forward—an act of mediation—motivates the story of survival, but mourning's sense of belatedness necessarily tinges the survivorhood of a reader charged with responding to the act of witness, requiring the response to become an act of relay in its turn. So a brief meditation on reading as a mode of mourning seems indicated, in part because we are not accustomed to considering reading, often thought to be a private act, in the context of social phenomena such as mourning, and in part because it is the dynamics of mourning and the inadequacy of readerly response that account for the relay character of reading in the chain of witness and require a reader to send the witnessing message forward in turn. By their literalization of the theoretical proposition summarized in the phrase "the death of the author," AIDS diaries require us in a quite particular sense to take seriously the model of reading as a mode of mourning, but the theoretical proposition itself implies a sense in which *all* reading—reading as a discursive event, not the purely linguistic act described by Barthes—must be tinged with mourning. The stress imposed on reading by its dependence on the author's death, whether theoretical or literal, is in my opinion a mark of that implication.

As was remarked in connection with Guibert (chap. 3), most academic theories of reading are theories of gain rather than loss. But loss is what mourning is about, and, if stressed reading is understandable as a mode of mourning, it is because the stress derives from a consciousness of loss. Unable either to retrieve an authorial subject who has died into the text or to actualize the full range of possibilities of textual signification that are released by the author's death, the reader experiences the anxiety of a double bind that would not arise were the author alive and had these responsibilities not become, as a consequence, readerly ones. In a readerly perspective the subject of *énoncé*, constructed differentially from the subject of enunciation (the *I* of "I am dying" as opposed to the *I* of "'I' is dead"), *may* be interpreted as being functionally equivalent to the (original) authorial subject, but this subject is inescapably an object of belated, readerly (re-)construction and offers no guarantee of authenticity, since—as Barthes might say—the text has become originless. On the other hand, however, real acts of reading, which are situated in a discursive economy (with its effects of power, desire, and knowledge through which we are constructed as persons, not pure subjectivities), cannot perform the role of the reader as it is mythically imagined—a purely linguistic agent of textual realization—in Barthes's essay. All readers thus function, in the end, something like critics (if not Barthesian Critics) to the extent that their consciousness of the problematics of authorial survival prevents their own sublimation into Barthesian readership. As anxious, mourning readers, they cannot and do not, Critic-like, reify an Author, since the authorial subject is construed as an effect of their interpretation; rather, they are conscious of their inability either to *wear* the author's sweater (as a gesture of simple continuation of the author's discourse) or to *ignore* the sweater—hanging relic-like on the coatrack and, as it were, "asking" to be worn—in the way that the Barthesian reader, participating in an act of substitution, is assumed able to do. In other words, the anxious reader, unlike the Barthesian reader but like the figure of Sid coming upon Andy's sweater, is a site of memory and subject to mourning.

Of course, a reader's memory of an author is not personal, like Sid's recall of Andy. It is a social memory, if I can so designate the sense in which collectivities can be conscious of the dead whom they have not known: conscious both of their loss and of their survival, their still active "presence" among those who survive them. And, in societies such as our own, there is a class of professional readers, called critics, who are specifically, if far from exclusively, charged with this function of social remembrance with respect to the dead authors in whom a living collectivity recognizes the members it has lost. From his authorial viewpoint Eric Michaels is right, then, to ask (as he does at one point, a bit sardonically—more tongue-in-cheek than with tongue provocatively extended): what can critics do? (157). Can criticism fight disease, save lives? Clearly not. But critics can mourn, and in addition they can participate in projects of witness. For critics are also, definitionally, readers who *write*, and their function is the production of commentary: that is, they produce texts that are, by definition, in a relation of some continuity with a prior text (without which commentary is meaningless) while nevertheless forming part of a genre that is specific and differentiating, having conventions of its own and regulating a mode of textual production in its own right. Because it belongs to the category of the "uptake," it is neither fully discontinuous nor fully continuous with prior texts (Freadman and Macdonald).

## RSVP, or Reading and Mourning

One might say, therefore—by way of an initial simplification—that the critic as reader is charged with a function of mourning, with respect to dead authors, while the critic as writer is in a position to furnish the relay function on which the continuation of witnessing projects, by virtue of their inevitably deferred character, depends. In both the mode of mourning and the mode of witnessing, criticism can thus be viewed as charged with significant responsibility for the afterlife of texts viewed as sites of discursive interchange, in which the death of an author requires both mourning for that death and continuation of the authorial project. I'll therefore take the figure of the critic as a model for an understanding of the mourning function of reading and of the witnessing function of writing when, in the mode of uptake, it relays a message marked by the authors' death and, like the CBC in Lynd's film, attempts to broadcast its effect.

For there is an ethics of criticism that forbids treating texts in cavalier or disrespectful fashion, as certain readers, for example, might take pleasure, or assert themselves, in "poaching," as Certeau puts it, on a text, appropriating it purely and simply for purposes of their own. (There is, of course, a postmodern celebration of reading as poaching, but it derives, I think, from a properly modest assessment of what a critical reader can do and is not inconsistent with the ethical position I have in mind.) This critical ethics puts the critic in exactly the double bind that I earlier described in terms of the requirement of responsiveness that is made of readers by texts whose authority derives from the death of the author. For it is understood as a particular responsibility of criticism to attempt to take account, in reading, of the context of a given text's historical production, a context readily conflated with the concept of the "author's sense" of a work. Whatever a critic's interest in producing contemporary relevance for a text grasped as an enunciation within the context of its reading, there is always a measure of historical, philological, and/or interpretive work that seeks to restore a putatively original sense through which the reading of contemporary relevance must pass even as it may differentiate itself with respect to it. A critic who did not acknowledge the pressure of such an "authorial" sense as part of a necessary respect for textual integrity would be an irresponsible critic. But the drama of criticism, if that is not too strong a word, derives both from the knowledge that the belated work of historical reconstruction is illusory (that the author is dead) and from the consciousness that contemporary meanings can only be produced not only differentially, with respect to those that are construed as having been once intended, but also as an actual *consequence,* therefore, of the author's death, from which critical commentary benefits because it derives its own authority from it.

There is thus an uncomfortable sense of exhuming—with difficulty and illusorily—an author, in the form of an authorial project, only to bury that author again, or that project, by making use of the resulting text to construct significations corresponding to the interests and purposes of the moment of reading. And it is the pressure of this immediate context of reading (it might include institutional contexts as well as changed historical circumstances) that not only sets critical authority against authorial authority but also prohibits the critic from fulfilling the task assigned by Barthes to his idealized reader, that of fully realizing the potential range of writerly significations released by the death of the author and the historical loss of an authorial project. As a discursive agent, a critic is thus inevitably positioned in innumerable ways that make the critic a double traitor, betraying both the author and the text the author's death has made possible. Tidy Town, as Eric Michaels might have said, always wins out, to the extent that the critic is charged with tidying out of the way those traces of an authorial project that seem no longer relevant to present concerns but also the full range of textual possibilities—possibilities that exceed the authorial project but which, also, cannot be made to fit the concerns of which the critic, in turn, is an agent. (Notice, as a case in point, the neat narratives constructed, thorough selective reading of a selected corpus, in this essay.) And this, then, is the mechanism whereby a deferred message, marked by the authors' death and received in the mode of (reading as) mourning, can only be continued—as, in particular, a project of witnessing requires—in the form of a new message.

One way of putting it (with a nod to *RSVP*) would be to say that a witnessing message that is received as "epitaph"—a genre in which the deceased putatively speaks to the passing wayfarer who temporarily survives—is passed on as "obituary," in which an other speaks, relaying the message of a dead person's life and work and doing so in sadness and love but only at the price of burying that per-

# RSVP, or Reading and Mourning

son with past-tense verbs and in the form of narrative closure.[3] It was while I was writing these paragraphs and pondering the epitaphic generic structure of Gautier's "Le spectre de la rose" (and its relation to obituary texts and death notices in *RSVP*) that I was invited—not, as it happens, a coincidence—to write an obituary for a very dear friend. Now, Gautier's rose employs a poet to give it a voice from the other side of death, much as Andy makes use of the CBC's request session for the same purpose. Such is the convention of epitaph:

Et sur l'albâtre où je repose
Un poëte avec un baiser
Ecrivit: Ci-gît une rose
Que tous les rois vont jalouser.

[And on the alabaster on which I lie
A poet, with a kiss,
Wrote: Here lies a rose
That every king will envy.]

The message is, of course, a deferred one, and the rose's death has intervened, but the discursive mode has the structure of "free indirect" style: the poet writes, but the thought (as when Flaubert puts us inside Emma Bovary's fictional mind) is assumed by the rose ("It is me that kings will envy"). On the other hand, the obituaries in *RSVP* are, by my count, three: in order of appearance, an obit we see being pinned up in the bookshop, the notice on a classroom door that is defaced with a huge scrawled word, *FAGGOT* (constituting a new message), and finally Andy's father's message to Sid, acknowledging Andy's and Sid's status as a couple: "I know how important you were

---

3. My scare quotes signal the functionality of these definitions within my argument. Epitaphs, as Reid (summarized in MacLachlan and Reid) has emphasized, cannot be defined in terms of any particular mode or structure of address, and Reid would probably want to say that "Le spectre de la rose" is a poem, not an epitaph. My point is that it is self-situated (MacLachlan and Reid would say intratextually framed) as an epitaphic poem, and, similarly, the death notice on the classroom door and the father's phone message are obituary-like rather than being obituaries. Finally, too, my argument hinges on the closeness of the epitaph and the obituary as genres—the continuity that permits a message received as epitaph to be sent on as obituary—as much as it acknowledges the discontinuity that I am stressing here.

to him." In their progression these three obituary instances aptly illustrate the degree to which obituary discourse buries the dead and substitutes for "their" message concerns, whether hateful or reconciliatory, which are those of the survivors. The free indirect structure that gave the rose a voice disappears from texts in which Andy no longer, in any sense, speaks. It was hard for me, therefore, to bring myself to write the obituary for my friend: the pressure for me to represent in some sense, that is, to bear witness to, the meaning of her life and the pressure to bury her in a neatly ordered narrative, the latter being the condition of the former, were each intense, and they were in irreconcilable conflict. But, in the end, I did it.

I did it, in the end—and however anxiously—because it would have been no easier for me to write an epitaph than to write her obituary. Once things are at the point where epitaphic and/or obituary genres become relevant, it is already too late. All witnessing discourse, including an author's original project, is definitionally deferred with respect to its object—that obscure *it* that it requires us to face—and the distinctions one tries to make, between message and response, sending and receiving, take and uptake, crumble in the face of the evidence of their equal inability to *say* what it is that they all, as acts of witness, invite us to face. In the way that a message is always already a response (always already deferred), a response (by definition deferred) is already always a message. The important thing, perhaps, is to recognize, as *RSVP* invites us to, that witnessing is a matter of forming chains of messages that are responses and of responses that are themselves messages, all marked by deferral, and that it is in those chains—in the act of relay, as an inadequate response to a message that was itself already inadequate, the act of transmitting it in hopelessly modified form—that the pain that is definitionally the object and motive force of witnessing discourse is inscribed. It is more important, then, for witnessing chains to be kept alive by acts of relay than for individual acts of representation to be judged (something they cannot be) accurate or even adequate.

No *message* is expressive of the pain. The pain lies—a readable object—in the fact of that inexpressivity, demonstrated as it is by chains of deferral to which it gives rise. The pain that discourse bears witness to is both the fact of discursive inadequacy in the face of pain and the fact that this discursive inadequacy fails to express. It is possible to write "I am dying" and to read "'I' is dead," but the message

## RSVP, or Reading and Mourning

"I am dead" (the burden of the rose's communication to its erstwhile wearer and of Andy's communication to Sid), although I who am living can write it, is one that cannot exist, either as a *literal statement* (one in which the signified, via reference, would be in undeferred relation to an actuality, such that the statement could not be read allegorically, like Andy's or the rose's) or as a *sincere utterance* (one in which *énoncé* and enunciation would be indistinguishable, such that neither "rhetorical" [intended] nor "dramatic" [unintended] irony would be inferred). We can range, on the "I am dying" side, writing like that of AIDS diaries, and on the "'I' is dead" side, reading as mourning and corresponding modes of mourning writing, like the epitaphic and the obituary. And with those discourses we pass *au plus près de la mort*, perhaps. But the unsayable, indescribable, inhuman *it* to which they bear witness comes within discursive range only to the extent that discourse, in the inadequacy of its deferrals, endlessly enacts its (*it's*) effects, gaining not the authority of death but one "borrowed," as Benjamin so cannily said, from death. We cannot know, understand, grasp, or comprehend, as long as we survive, what discourse is unable to say—but discourse, which has its own modes of survival, can teach us to face it.

The twentieth century, to those who have lived through it, feels like a period of unremitting pain. The two world wars, the two major revolutions (Russian and Chinese), the great depression, the Holocaust and nuclear fear, decolonization and the mass displacement of populations, the survival of historic oppressions and ancient hatreds, the cold war and the reversion of late capitalism, its historical competition apparently out of the way, to the ideology of laissez-faire and now a global epidemic, the effects of which might have been considerably mitigated were it not for government cynicism and social prejudice—all these, and others I haven't listed, have caused misery that has gone untold as well as provoking a mass of witnessing literature. There is probably an element of historical foreshortening in stressing the pain of the twentieth century, since, after all, humanity seems always to have been subject to war, famine, oppression, economic misery, gender and other violence, and epidemic. The practice of witness is also ancient: as old, at least, as the book of Exodus, it encompasses, for example, plague narratives and accounts of slavery. But, from the poetry and novels of the great war to the literature of the

Holocaust, the *testimonios* of Central America and the narratives and diaries of AIDS witness, our own century has indisputably seen an unprecedented surge in the production of witnessing texts.

This phenomenon raises at least two questions. One arises from the observation that not all emergencies produce witnessing texts and that each emergency seems to require the invention of its own forms of witness: there are conditions of possibility for the emergence of testimonial literature and determinants of genre that have not been theorized. Perhaps, in concentrating on the specificity of AIDS diaries, I will have made some slight contribution toward addressing that question, although ideally such a study should obviously be comparative. The second question asks why the twentieth century, unlike—or more so than—earlier periods, has been an age of witness. Here again there are conditions of possibility to consider. They include the greater access of oppressed, disadvantaged, and marginalized people to the means of self-representation: writing and other technologies of representation, publication and broadcasting, and so forth. They also include the failure of bourgeois comfort to protect the middle class, and notably its intellectuals, from the effects of war, ethnic and racial violence, pestilence, and the rest. But, if we look for an underlying motivation, a necessary cause deeper than the conditions of possibility, the clue lies, perhaps—this is a hypothesis for future work—in the characteristic orientation of practices of witness toward survival (living/dying to tell the tale) and the desire their structures of address imply for there to be a future. Our century might be the first period—or the first in a long time—to have seriously doubted the plausibility of humanity's having a future and to have turned to witnessing as a response to that doubt.

Witnessing, as a discursive genre, does not guarantee a future, of course. At most it foresees some sort of survival as an eventuality. If I am to survive in order to tell the tale, I must refuse the more obvious likelihood of my becoming a mere victim; if my tale is to survive me, it must find a future audience, and that audience must be responsive. What witnessing most profoundly bears witness to, then—over and above the horrors that it represents—is the desire for this to be the case: for me to survive or for my tale to find a reader. It cannot produce a future, but it can gesture in this way in the direction of that "after, after, after" that so wearies Derek Jarman but which nevertheless defines both personal survival and the survivorhood on which

## RSVP, or Reading and Mourning

textual survival depends. I've written this essay, therefore, and attempted to give some kind of "after" to the texts whose address structures I've responded to and whose message I've attempted to relay, because I share the desire that there be a future that I detect, as a reader, so poignantly at work not only in the texts but in the very fact of their having been written. It has been a work of mourning, and I hope a work of witness. But, reader, how will *you* respond? It's your turn now.

# Afterword

Having begun this essay in the summer of 1995, I am writing its afterword in the summer of 1997. During those two years the first vague rumors of the efficacy of protease inhibitors and the relative success of combination therapy began to spread and soon became real news. Problematic as this treatment is in many ways—medically, epidemiologically, and socially—it has bought valuable time for the unfortunately small number of people, relative to the magnitude of the world epidemic, who are in a position to benefit from it. In the group of Western, middle-class, usually white, gay men that has been largely responsible for the literature of AIDS witnessing, mortality rates have declined, and there is a certain sense of respite. The energy that for fifteen years went into anger and activism can be partially redirected into what for so long had to be deferred: mourning and the recognition of sadness. These emphases in my essay look like a sign, then, of the historical position from which it was written.

Some of the limits of its perspective come into focus, though, in the light of a diary that appeared in the fall of 1996, *Gary in Your Pocket*, a collection of writing by Gary Fisher—it includes poems and short stories as well as extracts from his voluminous diaries and accompanying notes—which was edited by Eve Kosofsky Sedgwick and thoughtfully presented, in a preface and afterword, by Don Belton and Sedgwick, respectively. Unlike the case of diary writers to whom an AIDS diagnosis may come as a unique catastrophe, Fisher's writing about AIDS is in absolute continuity with the difficulty in being— which is not the same as mere difficulty of being (in French I would say "difficulté à être," not "difficulté d'être")—that the whole diary records. Fisher was a black man brought up in a suburb surrounded by mainly white neighbors, whose sexual range included episodes entailing the enjoyment of humiliation and pain at the hands of, for preference, white partners, as well as practices that he knew were dangerous to his own and others' health. There is both a fierce affirmation of self in Fisher's writing and a certain surprise, even a bafflement or bewilderment, about his existence. AIDS aggravates but does not initiate what Sedgwick calls his "mutilated career" (278) and sees as constituting "a kind of allegory for the liminal" (276).

Resituating AIDS as part of a complex questioning of racial and sexual orthodoxies, Fisher's work also questions the assumptions I have shared with most of the authors in my corpus, then, in that he seems to have written, urgently, accurately, and voluminously but without much thought of publication or authorship. Both Belton and Sedgwick comment on his "diffidence" (285) and "ambivalence" (ix) in this respect. Concomitantly the scenario of posthumous textual survival consequent on the death of the author, which I have made my leitmotif, is absent from the texts of his that were, nevertheless published (thanks to the fortunate circumstance of his friendship with Eve Sedgwick). Gary Fisher had a need to write that was greater than his belief in being read. Political skepticism about the publishing industry played its role in this reticence. Don Belton quotes him as saying: "Where can a black, queer sociopath get a fair hearing anyway?" (ix). But, more profoundly, writing seems to have been important to him less as a way to ensure a "cultural future" than as present reassurance, as a way of giving a kind of substance and plausibility to life circumstances that must have seemed not just difficult but problematic and improbable. Thus, a character in one of his stories starts to keep a diary, "straining against her disbelief to be accurate," because she has been told that "once it's done . . . there's no way anyone, even you, can deny it happened" (110).

That same struggle, "against disbelief" and for accuracy, perhaps underlines the urgency with which Rafael Campo, in his remarkable memoir, "Fifteen Minutes after Gary Died" (in *The Poetry of Healing* [122–56]), describes Fisher filling up notebooks as he lay desperately ill in his hospital room. "The urgency of it all was in the tremulous handwriting, in the earthquake language, in the aftershock bloodstains" (138). Some of these hospital pages we can now read in print; even without the bloodstains they are like a free flow of direct, almost unmediated, subjective record, what he himself calls "a delirium of flashbacks and prayer and pressure drops and diarrhea . . . and dry heaves and waking nightmares and creeping skin and suicidal ten-

*Afterword*

dencies and unexpected and Poe-ish exponentials of hate and fear and fright, fantasy and fascination" (258). He was writing, in short, and, as he had said as early as 1989, "dying and writing this" (228), to save his life—but to do so in a number of possible senses. To save it, for example, through recording it, as one might save stamps or collect oddities, but to save it also, in the context of difficulty in being, by convincing himself through writing, and despite "suicidal tendencies" and other evidence of death wish, both of the reality of what was happening to him and of the strength of his desire to live. But finally, too, there is a sense he hints at parenthetically and tantalizingly, when he returns more skeptically, eighteen months later, to the thought that writing is self-rescue: "I wish writing could save my life (the way I may believe reading can)" (241).

This final, unexpected, concession that reading (in the sense of being read?) can be a form of life saving authorizes us then to think that, like writers more assured of publication and audience, Fisher must have found comfort in the thought that there would one day be a portable "Gary" whom readers could carry in their pocket, that a dying author can survive, in a certain sense, through the vehicle of readable text. And because it does, in the event, make Fisher's writing available for reading, *Gary in Your Pocket* finally does, therefore, ask the questions that are by now familiar to readers of this essay: what does it mean to read, and in reading to mourn the death of, an author whose dying of AIDS is recorded in a testimonial diary? To these questions Sedgwick, in her helpful and subtle afterword, gives answers consonant with what has been said here. "Gary" has been enclosed in a boxlike (coffinlike) container, but simultaneously—and here she relies on a poem by Whitman ("Whoever You Are Now Holding Me in Hand")—he has become, as no longer a writing subject but a subject of readability, "elusive." And furthermore, she points out, still making use of Whitman, this elusiveness is the sign of his continued resistance, a resistance that includes resistance to our reading and to our mourning because it is a turning away from those (still living) survivors in whom his own (posthumous) survival is invested.

If this is right, then Eric Michaels's rhetorical impudences may say something similar to what Gary Fisher's single-minded concentration on writing, as opposed to reading, might suggest or even the recurrent turning away from his reading audience that is implied by

Pascal de Duve's apostrophes to AIDS as "sida mon amour" in *Cargo Vie*. In certain forms of AIDS witnessing, the diary among them, the becoming-readable of the dying author can itself be given to us to read, and thus become interpretable, as a *withholding* of self—a withholding to which the act of publication does not give the lie so much as it confirms resistance to reading, the "withholding mode," as a desired and valid form of authorial survival. Thus Whitman:

> Even while you should think you have unquestionably
>     caught me, behold!
> Already you see I have escaped from you.

Gary Fisher's interest in writing rather than reading is one form of that authorial withholding, an ultimate way of producing readerly anxiety.

That said, however, when one reads *Gary in Your Pocket* in the context of combination therapy—thanks to which a fortunate few are beginning to be able to survive, in a less theoretical sense, a syndrome that continues, however, to kill millions and seems likely to do so into the foreseeable future—one is acutely conscious of the fact that Fisher's extraordinary writing might easily have remained obscure, gone unread because unpublished, and thus been denied access to the very elusiveness of readability I have just celebrated. It might have been, at best, a *Nachlass* or residue, comparable to the pathetic personal objects the dead leave behind them, sometimes to become props in memorializing practices (like Tom's eyeglasses in *Silverlake Life* or Andrew's sweater in *RSVP*), but often just to be given away or to become meaningless junk. In that sense, and in a way quite different from the *Nachlass* that is Barbedette's *Mémoires d'un jeune homme devenu vieux* (for Barbedette was a published author and only his reflections about AIDS were confined to unpublished jottings), *Gary in Your Pocket* speaks in a peculiar way for the countless numbers of those who in the epidemic have suffered but had no socially authorized voice, those without access to the privilege of writing, let alone the mechanics of publication—and for those, therefore, whom combination therapy and similarly expensive treatments will never reach and whom it is therefore imperative for the fortunate to remember, now, more than ever before. Even in a moment of respite, when it

## Afterword

becomes possible for some of us to acknowledge our sadness and indulge in our need to mourn, *Gary in Your Pocket* serves as a reminder both poignant and pointed that the time for activism and anger is still not over.

# References

Althusser, Louis. 1971. "Ideology and State Ideological Apparatuses." *Lenin and Philosophy and Other Essays*. London: New Left Books.
Apter, Emily. 1993. "Fantom Images: Hervé Guibert and the Writing of 'sida' in France." In *Writing AIDS: Gay Literature, Language and Analysis*, ed. Timothy F. Murphy and Suzanne Poirier, 83–87. New York: Columbia University Press.
Barbedette, Gilles. 1993. *Mémoires d'un jeune homme devenu vieux*. Paris: Gallimard.
Barthes, Roland. 1973. *Le plaisir du texte*. Paris: Editions du Seuil. Trans. Richard Miller as *The Pleasure of the Text*. New York: Hill and Wang, 1975.
———. 1984. "La mort de l'auteur." *Le bruissement de la langue*. Paris: Editions du Seuil. Trans. Stephen Heath as "The Death of the Author," in *Image, Music, Text*. New York: Hill and Wang, 1977.
Benjamin, Walter. 1969. "The Storyteller." In *Illuminations*, ed. H. Arendt. New York: Schocken.
Benveniste, Emile. 1974. (1966). *Problèmes de linguistique générale*. 2 vols. Paris: Gallimard.
Boulé, Jean-Pierre. 1995. "Hervé Guibert à la télévision: vérité et séduction." *Nottingham French Studies* 34, no. 1: 112–20.
Bowie, Malcolm. 1978. *Mallarmé and the Art of Being Difficult*. Cambridge: Cambridge University Press.
Brodkey, Harold. 1996. *This Wild Darkness: The Story of My Death*. New York: Metropolitan.
Buisine, Alain. 1995. "Le photographique plutôt que la photographie." *Nottingham French Studies* 34, no. 1: 32–41.
Campo, Rafael. 1997. *The Poetry of Healing: A Doctor's Education in Empathy, Identity and Desire*. New York and London: Norton.
de Certeau, Michel. 1990. *L'Invention du quotidien. 1. Arts de faire*. Paris: Gallimard (Coll. "Folio"). Trans. Steven Rendall as *The Practice of Everyday Life*. Berkeley: University of California Press, 1984.
Chambers, Ross. 1984. *Story and Situation: Narrative Seduction and the Power of Fiction*. Minneapolis: University of Minnesota Press.

## References

———. 1991. *Room for Maneuver: Reading (the) Oppositional (in) Narrative*. Chicago: University of Chicago Press.
———. 1993. *The Writing of Melancholy: Modes of Opposition in Early French Modernism*. Trans. Mary Trouille. Chicago: University of Chicago Press.
———. 1994. "Poaching and Pastiche." *Canadian Review of Comparative Literature / Revue Canadienne de Littérature Comparée* 21, nos. 1–2: 169–92.
———. 1997. "The Suicide Experiment: Hervé Guibert's AIDS Video *La pudeur ou l'impudeur*." *L'Esprit Créateur* 37, no. 3: 72–82.
Demme, Jonathan. 1993. *Philadelphia*. Videocassette. 125 min. Columbia Tristar.
Dresden, Sem. 1995. *Persecution, Extermination, Literature*. Toronto: University of Toronto Press.
Dreuilhe, Alain Emmanuel. 1987. *Corps à corps*. Paris: Gallimard. Trans. Linda Coverdale as *Mortal Embrace*. New York: Hill and Wang, 1988.
Duquénelle, Bertrand. 1993. *L'Aztèque*. Paris: Belfond.
de Duve, Pascal. 1993. *Cargo Vie*. Paris: Livre de Poche (Lattès).
Edelman, Lee. 1994. *Homographesis: Essays in Gay Literary and Cultural Theory*. New York and London: Routledge.
Felman, Shoshana, and Dori Laub. 1992. *Testimony: Crises of Witnessing in Literature, Psychoanalysis, and History*. New York and London: Routledge.
Fisher, Gary. 1996. *Gary in Your Pocket*. Ed. Eve Kosofsky Sedgwick. Durham: Duke University Press.
Frank, Felicia Miller. 1995. *The Mechanical Song: Woman, Voice and the Artificial in Nineteenth-Century French Narrative*. Stanford: Stanford University Press.
Freadman, Anne, and Amanda Macdonald. 1992. *What Is This Thing Called "Genre"?* Mount Nebo (Queensland): Boombana Publications.
Guibert, Hervé. 1981. *L'image fantôme*. Paris: Minuit. Trans. Robert Bononno as *Ghost Image*. Los Angeles: Sun and Moon, 1996.
———. 1982. *Les chiens*. Paris: Minuit.
———. 1986. *Mes parents*. Paris: Gallimard.
———. 1990. *A l'ami qui ne m'a pas sauvé la vie*. Paris: Gallimard (Coll. "Folio"). Trans. as *To the Friend Who Did Not Save My Life*. New York and London: High Risk / Serpent's Tail, 1994. (Translator unidentified.)
———. 1992. *La pudeur ou l'impudeur*. Videocassette. TF1. (Not commercially available.)
———. 1992a. *Cytomégalovirus. Journal d'hospitalisation*. Paris: Seuil.
———. 1992b. *L'homme au chapeau rouge*. Paris: Gallimard.
Halperin, David. 1995. *Saint Foucault: Towards a Gay Hagiography*. New York and Oxford: Oxford University Press.
Jarman, Derek. 1993. *At Your Own Risk*. Ed. Michael Christie. Woodstock, NY: Overlook Press.
———. 1994. *Modern Nature*. Woodstock, NY: Overlook Press.

# References

Johnston, Anna. Forthcoming. "Post Colonial Autobiography and Eric Michaels's *Unbecoming.*" *Meanjin.*
Joslin, Tom, and Peter Friedman. 1993. *Silverlake Life: The View from Here.* Videocassette. 99min. New Video.
Lynd, Laurie. 1994. "RSVP." In *Boy's Shorts.* Videocassette. 23 min. Frameline.
Lyotard, Jean-François. 1983. *Le Différend.* Paris: Minuit. Trans. Georges Van Den Abbeele as *The Differend. Phrases in Dispute.* Minneapolis: University of Minnesota Press, 1988.
———. 1988. *L'Inhumain. Causeries sur le temps.* Paris: Galilée. Trans. Geoffrey Bennington and Rachel Bowlby as *The Inhuman. Reflections on Time.* Stanford: Stanford University Press, 1991.
MacLachlan, Gale, and Ian Reid. 1994. *Framing and Interpretation.* Melbourne: Melbourne University Press.
Maclean, Marie. 1994. *The Name of the Mother: Writing Illegitimacy.* London and New York: Routledge.
Michaels, Eric. 1990. *Unbecoming.* Sydney: EM Press. (Rpt., Durham: Duke University Press, 1997.)
———. 1994. "For a Cultural Future: Francis Jupurrurla Makes TV at Yuendumu." In *Bad Aboriginal Art: Tradition, Media and Technological Horizons.* Minneapolis: University of Minnesota Press.
Monette, Paul. 1990. *Borrowed Time: An AIDS Memoir.* New York: Avon Books.
———. 1993. *Becoming a Man: Half a Life Story.* New York: HarperCollins.
———. 1994. *Last Watch of the Night.* San Diego: Harcourt Brace (Harvest).
Paulson, William. 1988. *The Noise of Culture: Literary Texts in an Age of Information.* Ithaca, NY: Cornell University Press.
Rudnick, Paul. 1994. *Jeffrey.* New York: Penguin.
Seckinger, Beverly, and Janet Jakobsen. 1997. "Love, Death and Videotape: *Silverlake Life.*" In *Between the Sheets, in the Streets: Queer, Lesbian, Gay Documentary.* Ed. Chris Holmlund and Cynthia Fuchs, 144–57. Minneapolis: University of Minnesota Press.
Sterne, Laurence. 1940. *The Life and Opinions of Tristram Shandy, Gentleman.* Indianapolis and New York: Odyssey Press (Bobbs-Merrill).
Taylor, Paul, ed. 1985. *Hysterical Tears: Juan Davila.* Richmond (Victoria): Greenhouse Publications.
Waldby, Cathy. 1992. "AIDS, Death and the Limits of Identity. Reading Eric Michaels's *Unbecoming.*" *Southern Review* 25, no. 2.
Wojnarowicz, David. 1991. *Close to the Knives: A Memoir of Disintegration.* New York: Vintage.